Atlas of Common Retinal Diseases in Nigerians

Second Edition

Tunji S. Oluleye MBBS, FWACS, FMCOPH, FVRS, FICO
Senior Lecturer & Consultant Ophthalmologist
University of Ibadan and University College Hospital, Ibadan

With contributions from:
Adekunle Rotimi Samuel MBBS, FWACS, FMCOPH
Lecturer & Consultant Ophthalmologist
University of Lagos & Lagos University Teaching Hospital, Lagos

BOOKBUILDERS ● EDITIONS AFRICA

ISBN: 978-978-921-208-8

Published in Nigeria by
BookBuilders • Editions Africa
2 Awosika Avenue, Bodija, Ibadan
www.bookbuilderseditionsafrica.org
email: folatundeus@yahoo.com;
bookbuildersafrica@gmail.com
mobile: 08068052154

CONTENTS

FOREWORD

It is my pleasure to write the foreword to this book titled *Atlas of Common Retinal Diseases in Nigerians*. At last, a pictorial book of retinal diseases in the tropics is a welcome development in our sub-region. We have depended long enough on retinal images of Caucasians eyes and so an atlas on retinal diseases in Nigerians is a dream come true.

Dr. T.S. Oluleye brings over 20 years expertise in ophthalmology and more than 10years expertise in the treatment of retinal diseases to bear in the publication of this book. Dr. Oluleye has a passion for teaching and when he brought up the new innovation of using IPhone with a +20D lens to take retinal pictures, he brought the teaching of difficult cases down to the level of the trainees for easy assessment and learning in a resource-limited setting like ours. The inclusion of some pertinent studies on retinal diseases has added more value to the book as it not only offers easy-to-understand pictures, but also offers some evidence from research work already carried out.

I therefore recommend this book to medical students and doctors-in-training who will find this book easy to refer to while in clinic to confirm the type of retinal disease their patients have. I also recommend this book to consultants who want to regularly refresh their knowledge about retinal diseases. The book is easy to understand with very clear pictures. I hope this effort by Dr. Oluleye will encourage other sub-specialties in ophthalmology to do the same and bring up pictorial books on our various sub-specialties.

Prof. Aderonke Baiyeroju
Department of Ophthalmology,
University of Ibadan,
Nigeria

PREFACE

The atlas of retinal diseases in Nigerians is long overdue. It is important to document common retinal diseases in Nigerians. This will enhance teaching, patient education and management of such diseases. The medical students and the postgraduate students will find the book useful as a quick reference. The general ophthalmologist will also find it useful as a diagnostic tool.

This book showcases some common retinal diseases in Nigerians seen at the retina clinics during a ten-year period of the author's post fellowship training at the University College Hospital, Ibadan and the Lagos University Teaching Hospital, Lagos. My colleague, Dr Rotimi–Samuel, a contributing author, also fell in love with the use of mobile phones for fundus photography. Over 90 percent of the retina pictures used in this book were taken with a mobile phone and a 20 diopter lens, a novel approach for taking fundus pictures in resource-poor settings of sub-Saharan Africa. A chapter of this book is dedicated to this method of retina examination which is set to overcome the challenges of fundus photography in the tropics. Some major retinal studies are also summarized to help in the management of some of these diseases.

ACKNOWLEDGMENT

I thank the Almighty God for the opportunity to put this work on paper. I also appreciate my co-author, Dr Rotimi–Samuel, who accommodated me at the Lagos University Teaching Hospital (LUTH) during my sabbatical leave. Some of the pictures were taken during this period. Drs Ajayi and Ilo are appreciated for their contributions.

I thank members of the Department of Ophthalmology, University College Hospital, Ibadan, for their support. I use this opportunity to thank my current Head of Department, Prof Ashaye, and the consultant staff for their encouragement. I also appreciate the ophthalmology residents for always challenging me to do more. To Prof Baiyeroju, who encouraged me into the retina sub-specialty, I thank you ma.

To my family, I thank you for the support. My father and mother, Pa Samuel Oluleye and Madam Dorcas Oluleye, I thank you for the gift of education. And to my siblings, I thank you all. To my immediate family, my lovely wife and sweetheart, Kehinde, thank you for your love and for supporting me all the way. My children, Temiloluwa, Olaoluwa and Modupe Ore-Oluwa, thank you for your love. I love you all. Finally, to the patients, who consented for their retina to be photographed, thank you.

Tunji S. Oluleye

To God be the glory for life and inspiration. I thank my Head of Department, Professor Akinshola, and the consultant staff of the Department of Ophthalmology, College of Medicine, University of Lagos, for their support. I also appreciate my residents and the entire members of staff of the Guinness Eye Center, LUTH, Lagos.

To Kate, my wife, and Omotara, Omowumi, Afolabi and Omololu, my children, I love you. I sincerely thank my parents, Late (Mr) Samuel Fagbemi and Mrs Fagbemi, for putting me on the right path of education.

Adekunle Rotimi-Samuel

One

Retinal Breaks & Retinal Detachment

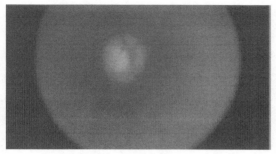

1.1. Posterior vitreous detachment (PVD).
Courtesy: Aravind.

Retinal Breaks (Tear/hole-full defect in retina)

Causes of retinal tear: Posterior vitreous detachment and trauma (blunt or penetrating) with vitreous incarceration (figures 1.1-1.7).

Causes of retinal holes: Atrophy, lattice, degeneration, myopia and connective tissue diseases such as Marfan's syndrome.

Treatment: Laser barrage on attached retina for symptomatic breaks; if retina is detached, retinal detachment surgery is indicated.[1]

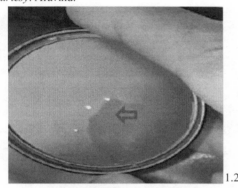

1.2

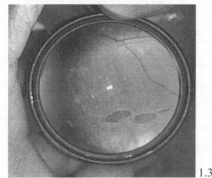

1.3

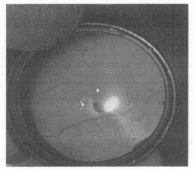

1.4. Retina hole, IOFB (PELLET) with retinal detachment.

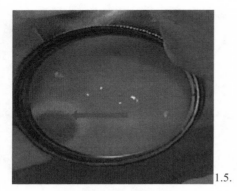

1.5.

Rolled edge of retinal hole and retinal detachment signifying long-standing condition.

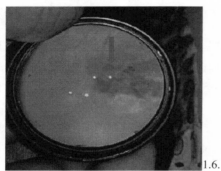

1.6.

Pigmented lattice degeneration with retinal hole (arrow). Laser barrage is recommended to prevent retinal detachment.

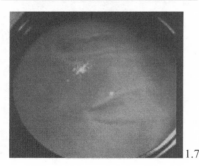

1.7

Symptomatic horse shoe retinal tears are as a result of posterior vitreous detachment and are precursors of rhegmatogenous retinal detachment. Urgent laser barrage is advised to prevent retinal detachment.[2]

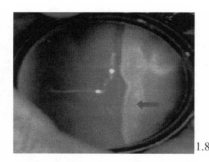

1.8

Giant retinal tear occurs where the tear is more than one quadrant. The edge of tear can roll (figure 1.9).

Treatment:

- Vitrectomy with silicone oil injection[3]
- Scleral buckle in selected cases

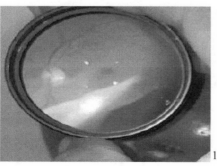

1.9

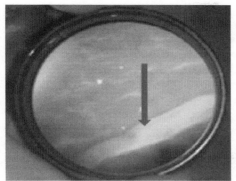

1.10. Retinal detachment and giant retinal tear with the rolled edge of the retinal tear.

Proliferative vitreoretinopathy can develop rapidly in giant retinal tears. Intervention is urgent.

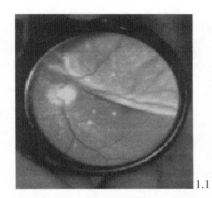

1.11

Superior retinal detachment can progress rapidly because of gravity. Urgent retinal detachment surgery is indicated to save the macula (figure 1.11). Figure 1.12 shows an inferior retinal detachment.

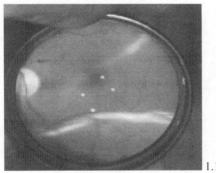

1.12

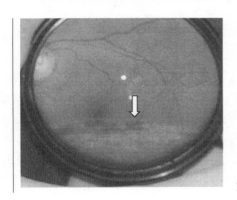

1.13.

Demarcation line (arrow) limiting the extension of an inferior retinal detachment into the macula.

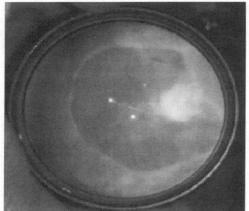

1.14. Tractional retinal detachment from proliferative diabetic retinopathy.

Fibrovascular proliferation in diabetic retinopathy causes tractional retinal detachment. Vitrectomy, membrane dissection and endo laser is advocated.

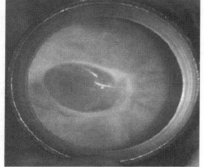

1.15. Tractional retinal detachment sparing the fovea.

Central vision may be preserved to some extent in patients with extramacular tractional detachment (figure 1.15).

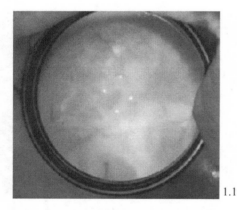

1.16

Advanced diabetic eye with severe tractional retinal detachment may still benefit from vitrectomy and membrane peeling.

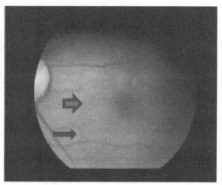

1.17

Exudative retinal detachment from central serous retinopathy (arrows showing the edge of serous detachment in figure 1.17). Treatment includes observation as spontaneous resolution is common. Focal laser to pigment epithelial detachment may help in non-resolving cases.[4]

Vogt- Koyanagi- Harada's disease (VKH)

This is a multisystem disease. Alopecia, vitiligo and poliosis occur as cutaneous manifestations. Bilateral exudative retinal detachment is a manifestation of the posterior uveitis associated with the syndrome. Systemic steroids and immunosuppressive treatment is advocated. Other features include headache, tinnitus and disc oedema.[5]

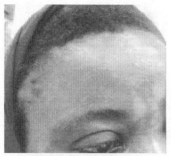

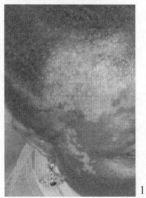

1.18

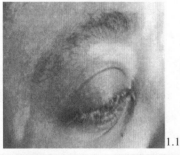

1.19

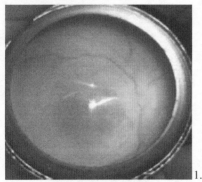

1.20

Bilateral optic disc oedema in the patient with VKH (figures 1.20 and 1.21).

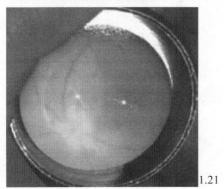

1.21

The patient also presented with bilateral exudative retinal detachment.

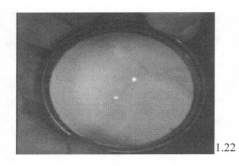

1.22

Exudative retinal detachment in both eyes of another patient with VKH (figures 1.22 and 1.23).

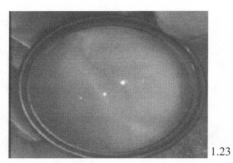

1.23

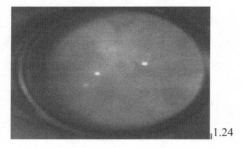

1.24

The same patient with VKH above after two weeks of systemic steroids with resolving detachment (figures 1.24 and 1.25).

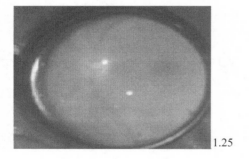

1.25

Two

Retinal Vascular Diseases

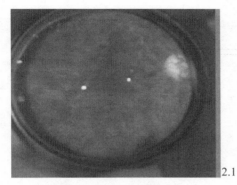

2.1

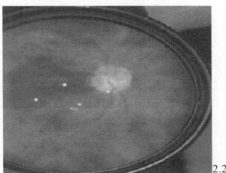

2.2

Retinal Vein Occlusion: Central retinal vein occlusion showing widespread retinal haemorrhage (figures 2.1 and 2.2). Risk factors include atherosclerosis, systemic hypertension, hypercoagulability state and raised intraocular pressure. Complications include macular oedema and neovascular glaucoma. Current treatment includes anti-VEGF injections for macular oedema and laser photocoagulation for neovascularization.[6,7]

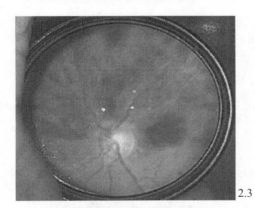

2.3

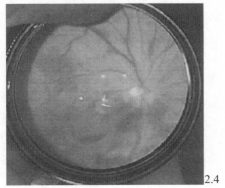

2.4

Hemi-Central Retinal Vein Occlusion: This is a variant of central retinal vein occlusion (superior HCRVO in figure 2.3 and inferior in figure 2.4). In HCRVO, separate veins drain the superior and inferior retina. Treatment is the same as for CRVO.

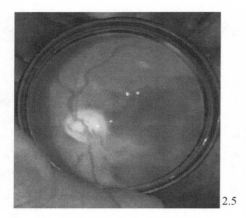

2.5

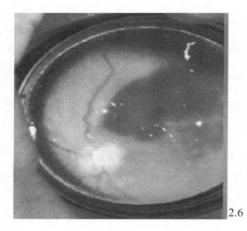

2.6

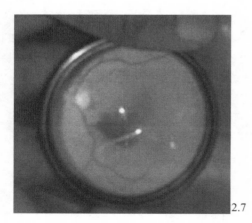

2.7

Branch Retinal Vein Occlusion: This occurs at arteriole venous crossing (figure 2.5: infero temporal BRVO, figure 2.6: supero temporal BRVO, figure 2.7: minor BRVO). Risk factors include systemic hypertension and raised intraocular pressure. Complications include macular oedema and retinal neovascularization with tractional retinal detachment. Treatment includes anti-VEGF, grid laser for macular oedema and sector pan retinal laser for new vessels. Vitrectomy is indicated for vitreous haemorrhage and tractional retinal detachment.[8-10]

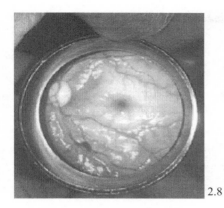

2.8

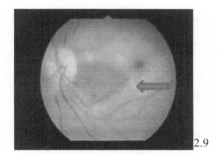

2.9

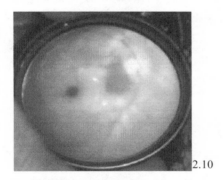

2.10

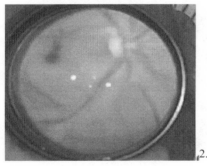

2.11

Retinal Artery Occlusion

Central retina artery occlusion presents with sudden painless loss of vision. Examination shows widespread retinal oedema with a macular red spot. Risk factors include embolization from valvular heart disease, systemic hypertension, diabetes and cholesterol emboli. Treatment include reduction of intraocular pressure, inhalation of carbogen, anterior chamber paracentesis, administration of blood thinners such as pentoxyphylin and ocular massage. Patient must present within 12 hours for any meaningful recovery of vision.[11] The cilioretinal artery may be spared as in figures 2.9 and 2.10. Central vision may still be good. In branch retina artery occlusion, visual field defect is seen.

Three

Diabetic Retinopathy

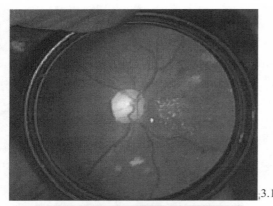

3.1

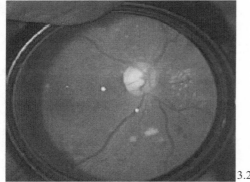

3.2

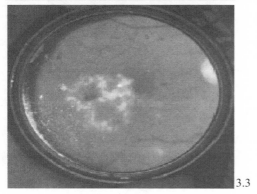

3.3

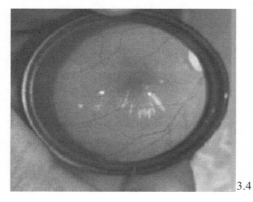

3.4

Diabetic mellitus produces microangiopathy in the eyes, leading to vascular occlusion, ischaemia, and release of vascular endothelial factors. Vascular leakage and neovascularization occur. The resulting retinopathy may lead to macular oedema/ischaemia, retinal and vitreous haemorrhage, tractional retinal detachment and neovascular glaucoma. Dot haemorrhages, hard exudates and cotton wool spots are signs of non-proliferative retinopathy. (figures 3.1 and 3.2). Circinate hard exudates cause macular oedema from leaking micro aneurisms. (figures 3.3 and 3.4). Treatment of non-proliferative diabetic retinopathy include control of systemic disease, anti-VEGF intravitreal injections for diabetic macular oedema and focal laser for clinically significant macular oedema (CSME).[12]

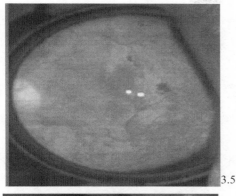

3.5

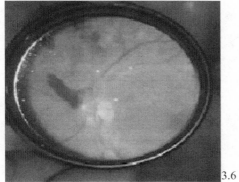

3.6

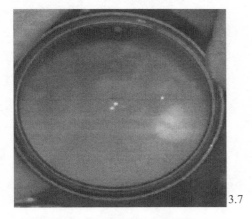

3.7

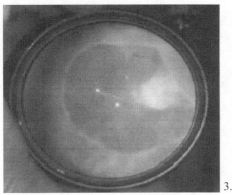

3.8

Proliferative Diabetic Retinopathy: This is characterized by new vessels on the disc or elsewhere (figure 3.5 and 3.6). They are prone to bleeding (figure 3.7). Treatment includes control of systemic disease and pan retinal laser photocoagulation. Recurrent bleeding from the fibrovascular proliferation may predispose to tractional retinal detachment (figure 3.8). Vitrectomy is recommended for vitreous haemorrhage and tractional retinal detachment.[12]

Four

Hypertensive Retinal Diseases

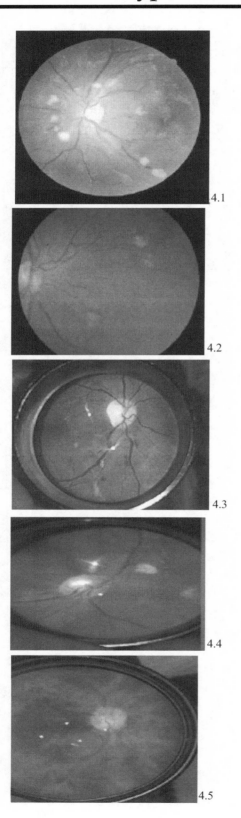

4.1

4.2

4.3

4.4

4.5

Systemic hypertension produces hypertensive retinopathy. Cotton wool spots, narrowing of arterioles, artero venous crossing changes and flame-shaped haemorrhage are features of hypertensive retinopathy. (figures 4.1-4.4) Systemic hypertension is a risk factor for retinal vascular occlusion (figure 4.5).[13]

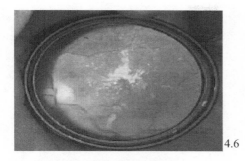

4.6

In pregnancy-induced hypertension (pre-eclampsia and eclampsia), choroidopathy produces exudation and macular star that resolves after delivery with control of the blood pressure (figure 4.6).

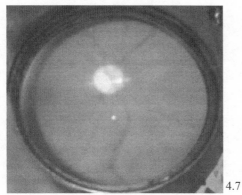

4.7

Hypertensive Optic Atrophy: This is a feature of systemic hypertension induced optic neuropathy.

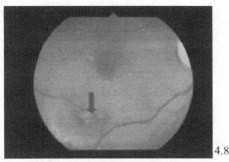

4.8

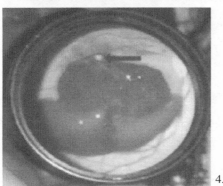

4.9

Retinal Arterial Macro Aneurism: This is a complication of systemic hypertension. Leakages from the aneurism may produce macular oedema (figure 4.8). Rupture of the aneurism may produce retinal and vitreous haemorrhage (figure 4.9). Treatment includes control of systemic hypertension, anti-VEGF and laser photocoagulation.[14]

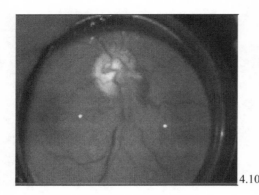

4.10

Anterior Ischaemic Optic Neuropathy: Non-arteritic with sectoral disc oedema. Control of systemic hypertension and steroid therapy may hasten resolution.

Five

Sickle Cell Retinopathy

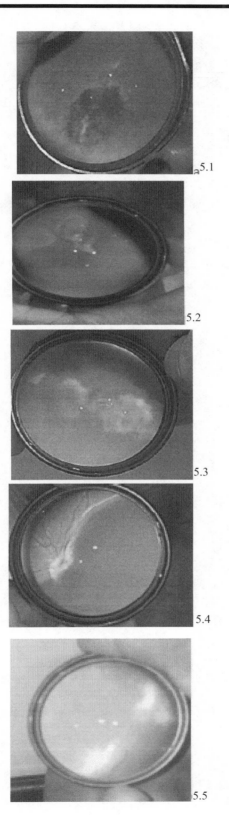

5.1

5.2

5.3

5.4

5.5

Haemoglobin SC Retinopathy: This is characterized by peripheral retinal ischaemia. Non-proliferative features include black sunburst which are retinal pigmentation reaction to retinal haemorrhage (figure 5.1). Proliferative features include new vessel formation, fibrovascular proliferation (sea fan) and recurrent vitreous haemorrhage (figures 5.2-5.4). Tractional retinal detachment may complicate retinopathy. Treatment with pan retinal laser photocoagulation applied to the retinal periphery may cause regression of the new vessels. Vitrectomy is recommended for persistent vitreous haemorrhage and tractional retinal detachment.[15]

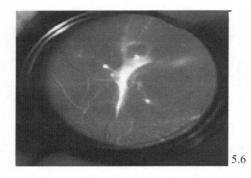

5.6

Retinal Vasculitis

Retinal vasculitis in young patients present as an idiopathic peripheral retinal vascular inflammation often associated with Koch's disease. The picture shows ghost peripheral vessels and regressed fibrovascular proliferation, indicating old resolved retinal vasculitis. Steroids is indicated in the acute phase, while laser photocoagulation can cause regression of new vessels.

Coats Disease

Coats disease is an idiopathic retinal vascular disease with telangiectasia and exudation. It is common in young patients and may be a close differential diagnosis of retinoblastoma (figures 5.7 and 5.8.). Treatment include anti-VEGF, laser photocoagulation, cryotherapy and scleral buckle surgery with or without vitrectomy.

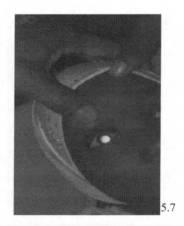

5.7

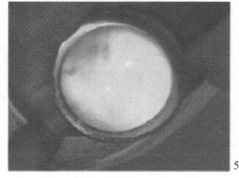

5.8

Six

Age-Related Maculopathy

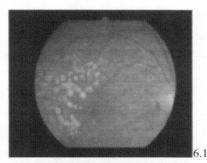

6.1

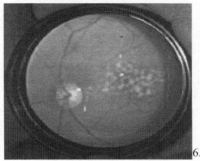

6.2

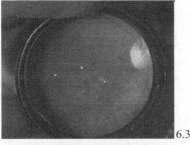

6.3

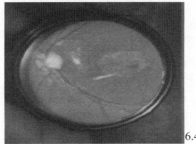

6.4

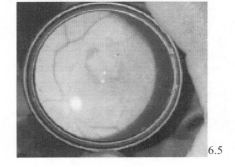

6.5

Age-Related Macular Degeneration (AMD)

Age-related macular degeneration is characterized by the presence of intermediate to large yellow sub-retinal deposits called soft drusens (figures 6.1 and 6.2).[16]

Advanced age-related maculopathy (ARM) could be dry age-related macular degeneration characterized by geographic atrophy (figures 6.3 and 6.4). Supplements of vitamin A (25,000IU), C (500mg), E (400IU), and minerals such as copper (2mg) and zinc (80mg) is beneficial.[17] Low vision aid is advocated for advanced stages.

Wet age-related macular degeneration is characterized by choroidal neovascular membrane (CNVM). Features of CNVM include macular haemorrhage, exudates and oedema or disciform scar in advanced stages (figures 6.5-6.7). Intravitreal anti-vascular endothelial growth factor is recommended.[18,19]

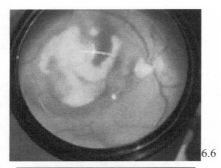

6.6

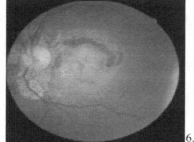

6.7

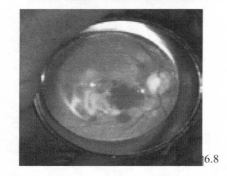

6.8

Wet AMD can lead to formation of macular scar from old choroidal neovascular membrane. Low vision aid is beneficial (figure 6.9).

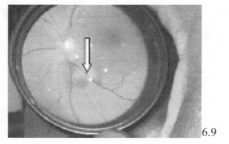

6.9

Haemorrhagic pigment epithelial detachment may be a part of AMD presentation or from idiopathic polypoidal choroidal vasculopathy (IPCV)(arrow). Anti-VEGF injection is recommended.

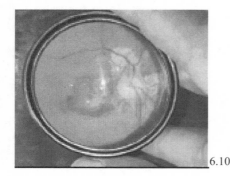

6.10

Seven

Idiopathic Polypoidal Choroidal Vasculopathy

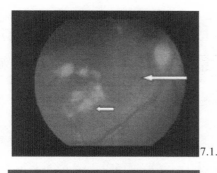

7.1.

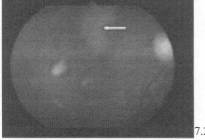

7.2

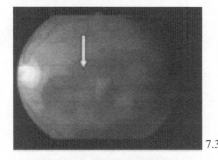

7.3

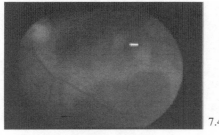

7.4

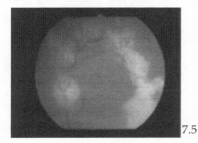

7.5

Idiopathic polypoidal choroidal vasculopathy (IPCV) was initially thought to be a variant of AMD, with abnormal choroidal vessels. Presentation occur in younger hypertensive women. Sub-retinal orange lesions (long arrow), exudates and haemorrhagic detachment of retina is characteristic of IPCV. Breakthrough vitreous haemorrhage is not uncommon. Sub-retinal haemorrhage from IPCV is shown in figures 7.3 and 7.4. Indocyanine green angiography (ICG) is helpful in the diagnosis of some challenging cases.[20] Treatment with antiVEGF and photodynamic therapy with laser may reduce symptoms.[21]

Exudates from idiopathic polypoidal choroidal vasculopathy is shown in figure 7.5.

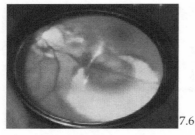

Sub-retinal haemorrhage from IPCV threatening the macula is shown in figure 7.6.

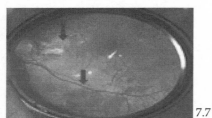

Same patient after treatment with anti-VEGF. Note the sub-retinal orange lesions (arrows) in figure 7.7.

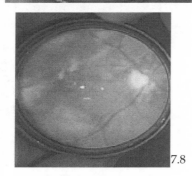

IPCV with sub-retinal orange lesions and retinal haemorrhage in the other eye of the patient in the previous picture is shown in figure 7.8.

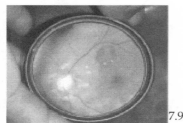

Recurrence in the left eye after 4 years.

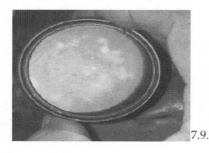

Scarred retina from IPCV.

Eight

Hereditary Retinal Diseases

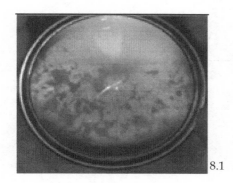

8.1

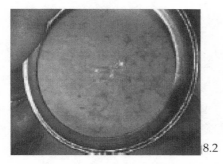

8.2

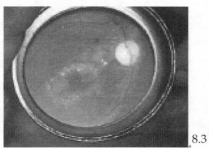

8.3

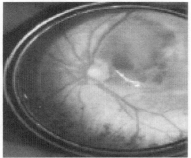

8.4. Retinitis pigmentosa with CNVM.

Retinitis pigmentosa is a hereditary degeneration of the retina involving the photoreceptors. Bone spickle retinal pigmentation (figures 8.1 and 8.2), attenuated retinal vessels and optic atrophy are common findings (figure 8.3). Cellophane maculopathy, cystoid macular oedema and atrophic maculopathy are common (figure 8.3). Choroidal neovascular membrane (CNVM) may be seen (figure 8.4). Treatment includes low vision aids, carbonic anhydrase inhibitor for macular oedema and cataract surgery for posterior sub-capsular cataract. Anti-VEGF is recommended for CNVM.

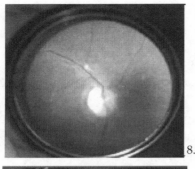

8.5

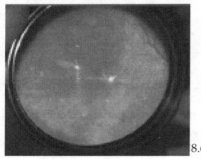

8.6.

Retinitis Punctata Albiscence: This is a variant of retinitis pigmentosa. Most authors believe it is an early stage of retinitis pigmentosa. It is characterized by the presence of whitish retina dots, attenuated retinal vessels, pale optic disc (figures 8.5 and 8.6) and poor night vision.

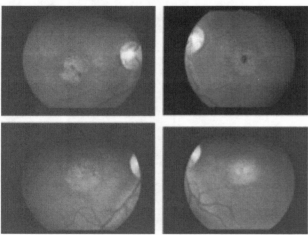

8.7. Stargardt's Disease

Stargardt's Disease: This is a form of hereditary macular degeneration. It starts in the first to second decade of life, with poor central vision. Fovea may be normal or show non-specific mottling, or with oval, 'snail-slime' or 'beaten bronze' foveal appearance, which may be surrounded by yellow-white flecks. Geographic atrophy may have a bull's eye configuration. Stem cell therapy is under consideration. The use of UV protective spectacles may reduce symptoms. Low vision aid is recommended.[22]

Yellow flecks surround the fovea in early stages of stargardt's disease.

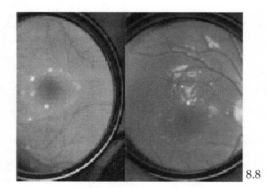

8.8

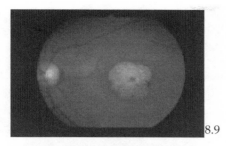

8.9

Geographic atrophy in the late stages of Stargardt's disease.

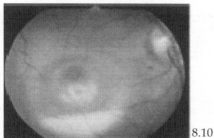

8.10

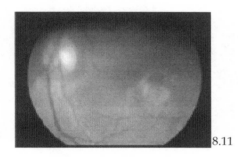

8.11

Best's Disease: This is also a form of hereditary macular degeneration. Figure 8.10 shows the pseudo-hypopyon stage of the disease, while figure 8.11 shows the atrophic stage. The disease starts in childhood, with a characteristic macular lesion resembling an egg yolk. It progresses through some stages before visual symptoms become apparent. The pathophysiology of Best's disease is explained by abnormality in the retinal pigment epithelium (RPE), with resultant abnormal ionic transport leading to the accumulation of lipofuscin in the RPE cells and sub-RPE space in the macular area. Degeneration of RPE cells can occur. Patients should be observed for signs of choroidal neovascular membrane treatable with anti-VEGF.[23]

Juvenile Retinoschisis

In a 12-year old boy with congenital retinoschisis, optical coherence tomography scan demonstrates the schisis cavities in the macula (figures 8.12 and 8.13) and Mitzuo reaction in the peripheral retina (figure 8.14). Topical and systemic carbonic anhydrase inhibitor may help reduce macular oedema.[24] Associated peripheral retinal retinoschisis may require laser and vitrectomy.

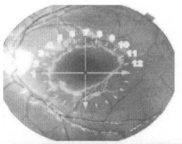

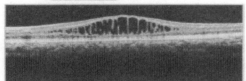

8.12

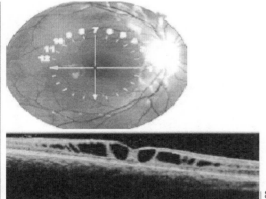

8.13

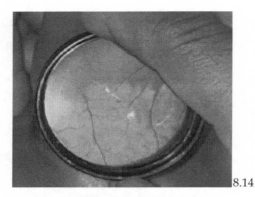

8.14

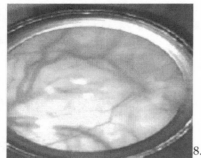

8.15

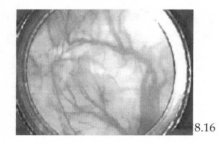

8.16

Albinism

Albinism is characterized by hypopigmented fundus, visible choroidal vessels, fovea hypoplasia and poor vision.

Low vision aid is recommended.

Nine

Toxic Retinopathy

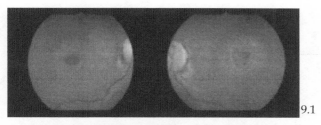

9.1

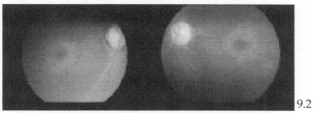

9.2

Chloroquine Retinopathy: This usually results from self-medication of chloroquine in Nigeria. Bull's eye manifestation comprising annular parafoveal chorioretinal atrophy have been described and is pathognomonic of chloroquine retinopathy (figure 9.1 and 9.2). The chloroquine accumulates in melanin of the retinal pigment epithelium.

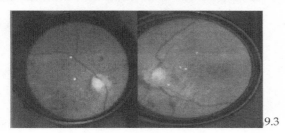

9.3

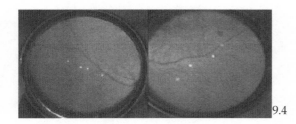

9.4

In addition to the bull's eye maculopathy, most patients with chloroquine retinopathy present with diffuse chorioretinal atrophy involving a large area of the posterior pole (figure 9.3), with a sharp demarcation between the posterior pole and the retinal periphery (figure 9.4).

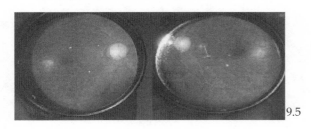

9.5

Chloroquine maculopathy with diffuse degeneration of the posterior pole with beaten bronze appearance of the macula is an advanced stage of the disease (figure 9.5).[25]

Ten

Macular Holes

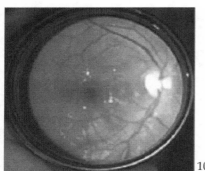

10.1

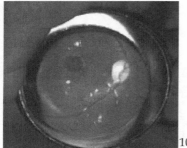

10.2

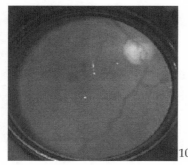

10.3

Risk factors include old age, myopia, blunt ocular trauma and solar retinopathy. The treatment recommended include vitrectomy, internal limiting membrane peeling with ILM flap inversion and intravitreal gas tamponade. Long-standing large macular hole may respond to treatment. Low vision aids may help.

Eleven

Valsalva Retinopathy

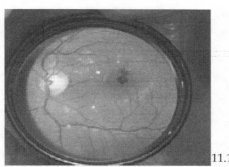

11.1

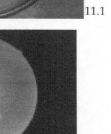

11.2

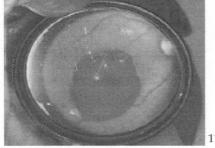

11.3

Risk factors include valsalva manouvers, systemic hypertension, constipation, cough, straining, labour and heated arguments. Rupture of the perifoveal vessels produces macular haemorrhage. Treatment is by observation. Spontaneous resolution occurs in most cases. Yag laser hyaloidotomy may hasten resolution in selected cases.

Twelve

Toxoplasma Chorio-Retinitis

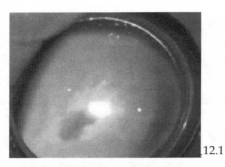

12.1

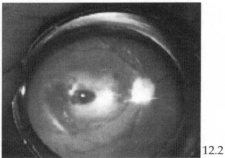

12.2

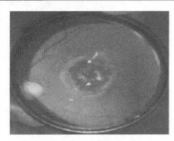

12.3

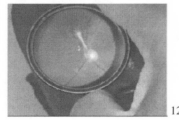

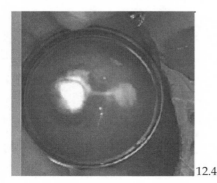

12.4

Toxoplasmosis

Retinochoroiditis or chorio-retinitis with an old pigmented scar and adjascent active retinitis is shown (figure 12.1 and 12.2). The patient presents with blurred vision from vitritis and retinitis if the optic nerve, macula and papillomacular bundle is involved. Treatment with pyrimethamine and sulphonamides is recommended.

Macur scar from congenital toxoplasmosis presents with a quiet lesion and no inflammation (figures 12.3 and 12.4)

Thirteen

Toxocara Retinal Granuloma

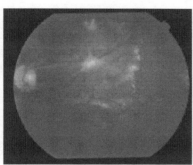

13.1. Toxocara retinitis scar.
Courtesy: Dr(Mrs) Ajayi.

Toxocariasis

This is toxocara granuloma with epiretinal membrane on the macula. It is common in children, adolescents and young adults. About 50% of the cases occur in the peripheral retina. Active lesion will benefit from antihelminthics and steroids. Quiet cases associated with epiretinal membrane will require vitrectomy and membrane peeling.

Fourteen

Tuberculous Retinitis

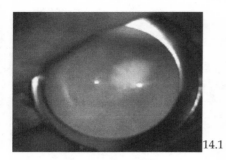
14.1

Ocular Tuberculosis

Ocular tuberculosis is characterized by choroidal granuloma (figure 14.1), retina abscess and chronic uveitis (figure 14.2). Ocular tuberculosis may occur without systemic or pulmonary manifestation. Treatment is as for pulmonary tuberculosis with multi-drug agents for 1 year.[26]

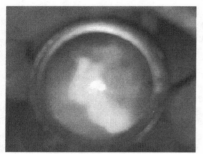
14.2. TB choroiditis with abscess

Fifteen

Cytomegalovirus Retinitis

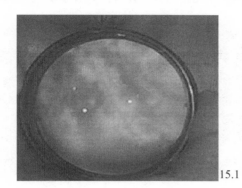

15.1

Cytomegalovirus retinitis is a marker for HIV infection and is characterized by retinitis exudates mixed with blood. It may show a granular appearance. First line therapy is oral valganciclovir. Patient should also be on HAART.

Sixteen

Retinopathy of Prematurity

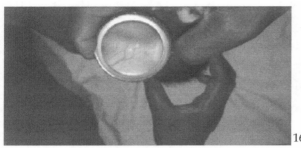

16.1

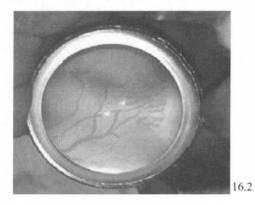

16.2

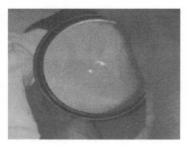

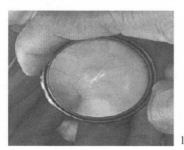

16.3

Preterm with low birth weight exposed to oxygen are at risk and should be screened. Figure 16.1 shows a mobile phone screenshot of the retina during screening. Mobile phone screening is being investigated for screening in poor resource settings of Africa.[27] Figure 16.2 shows peripheral retina showing a ridge with new vessels behind the ridge. Figure 16.3 shows the demarcation between vascular and avascular retina with retina haemorrhage in figure 16.4. Cryotherapy and laser treatment are recommended, with laser being preferred as no anesthesia is required.[28] Anti-VEGF is an emerging treatment proven to be better than laser.[29] Figure 16.5 shows bilateral advanced stage with bilateral retinal detachment — retrolental fibroplasia.

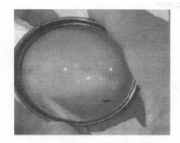

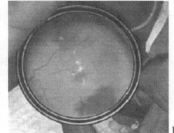

16.4

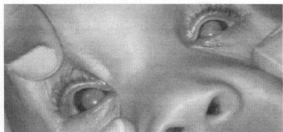

16.5

Seventeen

Retinal Trauma

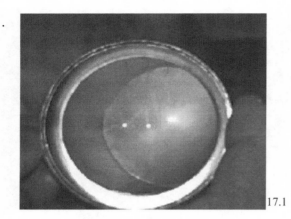

17.1

This involves a lens drop/traumatic lens dislocation into the vitreous cavity. Lens lying on the retina may produce retinal damage. Treatment include vitrectomy and lensectomy

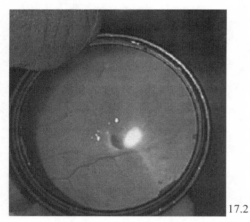

17.2

Traumatic retinal detachment from a gun/blast pellet creating a retinal hole. The pellet is under the retina. Vitrectomy, foreign body removal, laser retinopexy and silicone oil injection is advocated. Figure 17.3 shows multiple retinal tears from ocular blunt injury. Laser retinopexy is required to prevent retinal detachment.

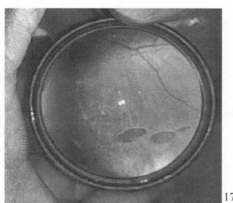

17.3

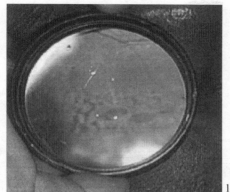

17.4

Same patient after laser barrage retinopexy (figure 17.4).

Eighteen

Retinal Malformations & Miscellaneous Lesions

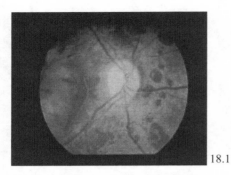

18.1

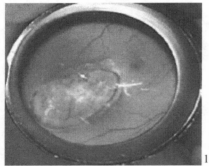

18.2

Retinochoroidal Coloboma: This results from incomplete closure of the optic fissure. Complications include rhegmatogenous retinal detachment. Treatment include laser barrage of the edge of the coloboma to prevent retinal detachment.

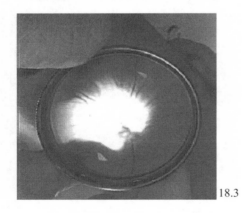

18.3

Myelinated Nerve Fibre: This is a benign condition and may regress spontaneously. Myelination usually should regresses before birth. Vision is usually not affected.

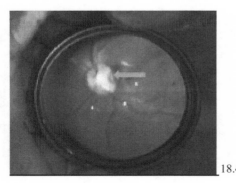

18.4

Optic Disc Pit and Macular Detachment: Optic pit is a congenital failure of closure of the terminal optic fissure. The pit is located at the temporal disc margin (arrow). A defect at the diaphanous tissue over the pit is responsible for macular detachment. Treatment include barrage laser and vitrectomy.[30]

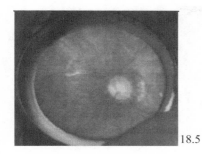

18.5

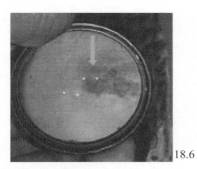

18.6

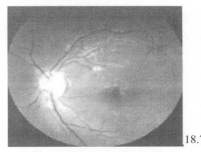

18.7

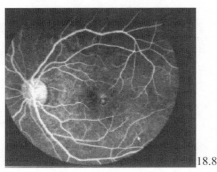

18.8

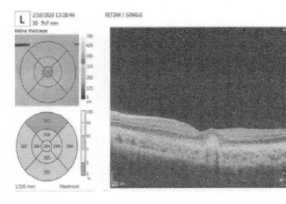

18.9

High Myopia: This is associated with fundus degenerative changes. Myopic crescents, retinal atrophy and peripheral retinal degenerations are common. Figure 18.6 shows a pigmented lattice with a retinal hole (arrow). Laser barrage is advocated to seal retinal hole.

Myopic Choroidal Neovascular Membrane (CNVM): This is associated with the development of a break in the Bruchs membrane under the fovea resulting in the ingrowth of choroidal new vessles. Patients present with sudden loss of central vision. Flourescein angiography shows classic choroidal new vessel at the fovea. Optical coherence tomography shows elevation of the RPE with the CNVM (figures 18.7-18.9) Treatment with intravitreal antiVEGF is beneficial.[31]

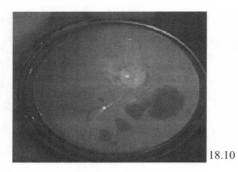

18.10

Congenital hypertrophy of the retinal pigment epithelium, also known as bear track pigmentation, is a benign condition that may grow slowly. Observation is advised.

Nineteen

Melanocytoma

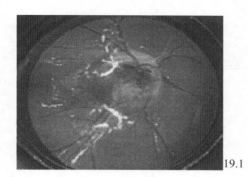

Optic Disc Melanocytoma: This is a benign pigmented optic nerve lesion arising from the melanocytes. It is common among dark-skinned individuals. Close monitoring is required to detect complications such as choroidal new vessels and serous detachment amenable to treatment.[32]

19.1

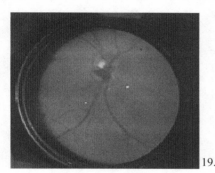

19.2

Twenty

Retinal Changes Associated
With Chronic Renal Failure

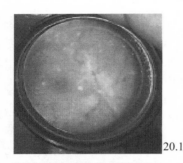

20.1

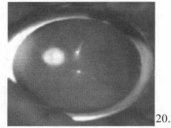

20.2

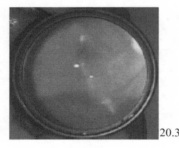

20.3

These pictures are from patients with chronic renal failure on dialysis. Signs of hypertensive retinopathy, choroidopathy and optic neuropathy are common findings, such as retinal oedema, attenuation of arterioles, optic atrophy (figure 20.1 and 20.2), silver wiring (figure 20.2), retinal ischaemia, neovascularization and vitreous haemorrhage (figure 20.3). Other findings include macular oedema and cotton wool spots (figure 20.1).

Twenty-One

Leukemia

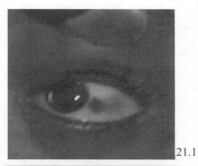

21.1

Subconjunctiva haemorrhage is a common manifestation of leukemia. The condition should be suspected in cases of subconjuctiva haemorrhage.

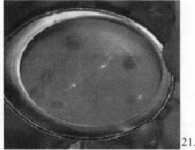

21.2

Multiple Roth's spots in the retina is common in leukemia. The retinal vessels are tortuous and dilated. Other features include disc oedema, infiltration and vitreous haemorrhage.[33]

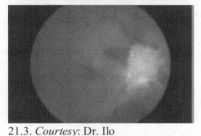

21.3. *Courtesy*: Dr. Ilo

Optic disc infiltration and oedema in patients with leukemia.

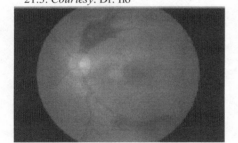

21.4. *Courtesy:* Dr. Ilo.

Retinal haemorrhage in leukemia.

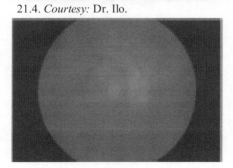

21.5. *Courtesy*: Dr. Ilo

Management of vitreous haemorrhage in patients with leukemia include control of systemic disease and use of anti-VEGF for proliferative retinopathy.

Twenty-Two

Tumour Secondaries

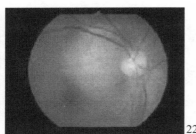

22.1

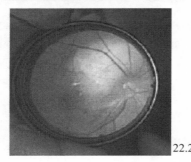
22.2

Secondaries from breast, prostate and lungs are common. Figures 22.1 and 22.2 are from a 56-year-old individual with a lung carcinoma. Chemotherapy to the primary tumour is advocated.

References

1. AAO. Posterior Vitreous Detachment, Retinal Breaks, and Lattice Degeneration. American Academy of Ophthalmology, San Francisco, CA, 2014.

2. Davis MD. Natural history of retinal breaks without detachment. *Arch Ophthalmol* 1974; 92:183-94.

3. Shunmugam M, Ang GS, Lois N. Giant retinal tears. *Survey of Ophthalmology* ,2014; 59(2): 192 – 216.

4. Abouammoh MA. Advances in the treatment of central serous chorioretinopathy. *Saudi Journal of Ophthalmology* 2015; 29(4):278-286.

5. Oluleye TS, Rotimi-Samuel AO, Adenekan A, Ilo OT, et al, Two cases of Vogt-Koyanagi-Harada's disease in sub-Saharan Africa. *Int Med Case Rep J.* 2016; 9: 373-376.

6. Heier JS, Campochiaro PA, Yau L, Li Z, Saroj N, Rubio RG, et al. Ranibizumab for macular edema due to retinal vein occlusions: Long-term follow-up in the HORIZON trial. *Ophthalmology* 2012; 119(4):802-9.

7. Central Vein Occlusion Study Group. A randomized clinical trial of early panretinal photocoagulation for ischemic central vein occlusion. The Central Vein Occlusion Study Group N report. *Ophthalmology* 1995; 102(10):1434-44.

8. Campochiaro PA, Sophie R, Pearlman J, Brown DM, Boyer DS, Heier JS. Long-term outcomes in patients with retinal vein occlusion treated with ranibizumab: The RETAIN study. *Ophthalmology* 2014; 121(1): 209-19.

9. Arnarsson A, Stefansson E. Laser treatment and the mechanism of edema reduction in branch retinal vein occlusion. *Invest Ophthalmol Vis Sci.* 2000; 41(3): 877-9.

10. Ikuno Y, Ikeda T, Sato Y, Tano Y. Tractional retinal detachment after branch retinal vein occlusion. Influence of disc neovascularization on the outcome of vitreous surgery. *Ophthalmology* 1998; 105(3): 417-23.

11. Pielen A, Pantenburg S, Schmoor C, Schumacher M, Feltgen N, Junker B, et al. Predictors of prognosis and treatment outcome in central retinal artery occlusion: Local intra-arterial fibrinolysis vs. conservative treatment. *Neuroradiology* 2015; 57(10): 1055-62.

12. AAO. Diabetic Retinopathy Preferred Practice Pattern. American Academy of Ophthalmology, San Francisco, CA, 2016.

13. Oluleye ST, Olusanya BA, Adeoye AM. Retinal vascular changes in hypertensive patients in Ibadan, sub-Saharan Africa. *International Journal of General Medicine* 2016; 9:285-290.

14. Speilburg, AM, Klemencic SA. Ruptured retinal arterial macroaneurysm: Diagnosis and management. *Journal of Optometry* 2014; 7(3): 131–137.

15. Oluleye TS. Pattern of presentation of sickle cell retinopathy in Ibadan. *J Clinic Experiment Ophthalmol* 2012; 3: 257.

16. Oluleye, TS. Age-related macular degeneration: Current concepts in pathogenesis and management. *Nig. J. Oph.* 2008; 16(1): 5-11.

17. Age-Related Eye Disease Study Research Group. A randomized, placebo-controlled, clinical trial of high-dose supplementation with vitamins C and E, beta carotene, and zinc for age-related macular degeneration and vision loss: AREDS report no. 8. *Arch Ophthalmol.* 2001; 119(10): 1417-36.

18.   Brown DM, Kaiser PK, Michels M, Soubrane G, Heier JS, Kim RY, Sy JP, Schneider S, ANCHOR Study Group. Ranibizumab versus verteporfin for neovascular age-related macular degeneration. *N Engl J Med*. 2006; 355(14):1432-44.

19.   Rosenfeld PJ, Brown DM, Heier JS, Boyer DS, Kaiser PK, Chung CY, Kim RY, et al. Ranibizumab for neovascular age-related macular degeneration. *N Engl J Med* 2006; 355:1419-1431.

20.   Oluleye TS, Babalola Y. Pattern of presentation of idiopathic polypoidal choroidal vasculopathy in Ibadan, Sub Sahara Africa. *Clinical Ophthalmology* 2013; 7: 1373-6.

21.   Yannuzzi L, Sorenso J, Spaide R, Lipson B. Idiopathic polypoidal choroidal vasculopathy (IPCV). *Retina* 1990; 10(1): 1-8.

22.   Oluleye TS, Aina AS, Sarimiye TF, Olaniyan SI. Stagardt's disease in 2 Nigerian siblings. *International Medical Case Report Journal* 2013; 6: 13-15.

23.   Oluleye TS. Best macular dystrophy in a Nigerian: A case report. *Case Rep Ophthalmol* 2012; 3: 205–208.

24.   Ghajarnia M, Gorin MB. Acetazolamide in the treatment of X-linked retinoschisis maculopathy. *Arch Ophthalmol*. 2007; 125(4): 571-3.

25.   Oluleye TS, Babalola Y, Ijaduola M. Chloroquine retinopathy: Pattern of presentation in Ibadan. *Eye (Lond)* 2016; 30(1): 64-7.

26.   Oluleye TS. Tuberculous uveitis. *Journal of Multidisciplinary Healthcare* 2013; 6: 41-3.

27.   Oluleye TS, Rotimi-Samuel A, Adenekan A. Mobile phones for retinopathy of prematurity screening in Lagos, Nigeria, sub-Saharan Africa. *Eur J Ophthalmol*. 2016; 26(1): 92-4.

28.   Shalev B, Farr AK, Repka MX. Randomized comparison of diode laser photocoagulation versus cryotherapy for threshold retinopathy of prematurity: Seven-year outcome. *Am J Ophthalmol*. 2001; 132(1): 76-80 .

29.   Mintz-Hittner HA, Kuffel RR. Intravitreal injection of bevacizumab (avastin) for treatment of stage 3 retinopathy of prematurity in zone I or posterior zone II. *Retina* 2008; 28(6): 831-8.

30.   Moisseiev E, Moisseiev J, Loewenstein A. Optic disc pit maculopathy: When and how to treat? A review of the pathogenesis and treatment options. *International Journal of Retina and Vitreous*, 2015, 1: 13.

31.   Ugalahi MO, Adeyemo AO, Ezichi EI, Olusanya BA, Oluleye TS. Presumed optic disc melanocytoma in a young Nigerian: A diagnostic challenge. *Nigerian Journal of Ophthalmology* 2016; 24(1): 46-48 .

32.   Sharma T, Grewal J, Gupta S, Murray P. Ophthalmic manifestations of acute leukaemias: The ophthalmologist's role. *Eye* 2004; 18: 663–672.

Mobile Phones for Fundus Photography

Introduction

The need to capture the image of the retina for teaching, patient education and monitor response to treatment is increasing. Unfortunately, the cost of a standard retina camera is beyond the reach of doctors in the developing countries of Sub- Sahara Africa.

The field of view of the direct ophthalmoscope is limited to about 5 degrees. Most physicians are reluctant to use it and patient education is not possible with it as only the doctor sees the retina. The indirect ophthalmoscope provides a wider field of view and helps in the examination of the peripheral retina. However, it has a difficult learning curve and too bulky for the general physician. Subsequently, mirrors were attached to the indirect ophthalmoscope to provide a teaching platform. Still, patient education was limited to retinal drawings and sketches made by the doctor. Many years later, video camera attachment to the indirect ophthalmoscope was developed. This improved teaching and patient education. The equipment came at a price not affordable to physicians in the poor resource countries. The fundus camera was later developed. It is bulky and the cost was too high for physicians in the developing countries. Attempts were made to develop a portable fundus camera. The available ones are still expensive for physicians in sub-Saharan Africa. Recently, portable devices such as the iexaminer in which the iPhone was attached to the panfundoscope were developed.[1] The device, though less expensive and portable, still has a sub-optimal field of view. Other devices were developed with a similar field of view.

Recently, workers at Massachusetts published their work on the use of iPhone and the 20D lens to capture retinal images likened to an indirect ophthalmoscope.[2] The field of view was satisfactory and the iPhone 5 produced an image with a good resolution, comparable to the conventional fundus camera. The workers recommended the use of an application (Filmic pro) to stabilize the image and reduce glare. They recommended the device for developing nations with poor resources. It is cheaper and more portable than the conventional fundus camera and can be used in developing nations for telemedicine, where images can be uploaded to email by resident doctors, physicians and GPs. The fundus pictures can be sent via email to ophthalmologists for review and suggestions concerning management. This method of retina imaging has been reviewed and found to be satisfactory.[3-5]

Techniques

The filmic pro app is launched with the continuous illumination of the camera flash set to the lowest possible level to reduce glare. The examiner holds the 20D lens with his dominant hand and the phone in the other hand. The flash of the mobile phone produces the illumination. The setup is used as a binocular indirect ophthalmoscope. The eye of the patient, the 20D lens and the flash/camera of the mobile phone must be on the same axis. The 20D lens captures the image of the retina, which is viewed by the examiner on the screen of the mobile phone (figure 23.1). The video recording mode is activated to capture the video of the retina examination. After the examination, using the iPhone editing software, still images or frames can be captured with a snapshot and saved into the picture gallery of the mobile phone for editing (figure 23.2-23.4).

For the Android phone, the application, Cinema FV 5, is available for download at the Google play store. Setting the illumination at the lowest possible level, video recordings of the retinal examination is possible as earlier described for the Iphone system. With the 20D lens, the set-up is used similarly as an indirect ophthalmoscope. An application, video to picture app from the Google play store is used to extract selected frames. The selected frames are edited as above. Alternatively, the applications may be bypassed by pasting a paper tape over the camera flash thereby reducing the illumination.

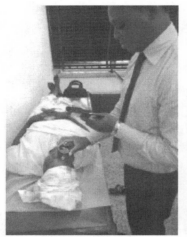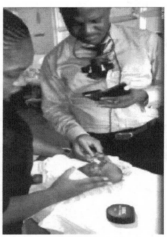

23.1. Techniques of using mobile phones to capture retinal images.

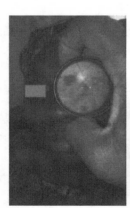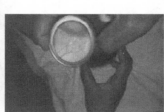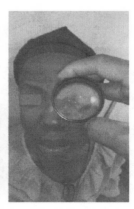

23.2. Screen shots of the mobile phone.

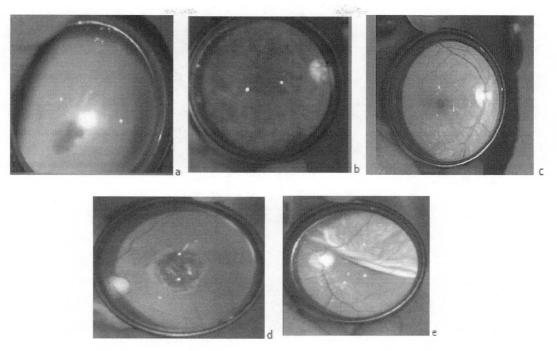

23.3. Edited pictures from the screen shot of Iphone: a, toxoplasmosis with retinochoroiditis; b, central retina vein occlusion; c, macular hole; d, macular scar; e, superior retinal detachment.

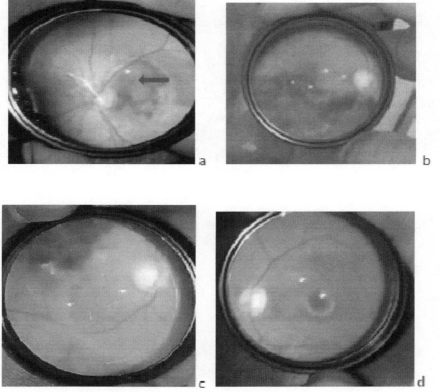

23.4. Edited pictures from Android phone: a, choroidal neovascular membrane (active); b, hemicentral retinal vein occlusion; c, supero temporal retinal vein occlusion; d, macular hole

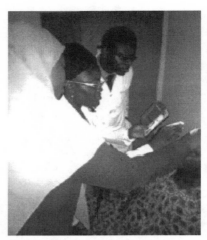

23.5. Doctors learning the method

References

1.   Welch Allyn. Iexaminer. www.welchallyn.com/en/microsites/iexaminer.html (Accessed on 3 July 2014).

2.   Haddock LJ, Kim DY, Mukai S. Simple, inexpensive technique for high-quality smartphone fundus photography in human and animal eyes. *Journal of Ophthalmology* 2013.

3.   Lord RK, Shah VA, San Filippo AN, Krishna R. Novel uses of smart phones in ophthalmology. *Ophthalmology* 2010; 117(6):1274-1274.

4.   Mahesh P, Divyansh KC, Madhukumar R, Rajesh R, Srinivasulu Y, Rodrigues G. Fundus imaging with a mobile phone: A review of techniques. *Indian J Ophthalmol.* 2014; 62(9): 960–962.

5.   Raju B, Raju N. Regarding fundus imaging with a mobile phone: A review of techniques. *Indian J Ophthalmol* 2015; 63:170-1.

Major Retinal Studies

A.   United Kingdom Prospective Diabetes Study (UKPDS)

Aim of study: To determine the effect of tight blood glucose control and blood pressure on diabetic retinopathy.

Study design: Prospective, multi-centre, randomized controlled trial.

Results: The study compared the intensive treatment with the conventional treatment. After 12 years of follow-up, diabetic retinopathy progression was reduced by 21% in the intensive group when compared with the conventional group. Likewise, the need for laser photocoagulation was also reduced by 29% in the intensive versus the conventional treatment group. After about 8 years of follow up, the group of patients in the tight control group had a 34% reduction in progression of retinopathy and a 47% reduced risk of deterioration in visual acuity of three lines compared with the less tight control group.

Importance of study: The UKPDS was a landmark trial in establishing the importance of both good glycaemic control and good blood pressure control in reducing the progression of diabetic retinopathy in patients with type 2 diabetes

References

1.   UK Prospective Diabetes Study (UKPDS) Group. Intensive blood-glucose control with sulphonylureas or insulin compared with conventional treatment and risk of complications in patients with type 2 diabetes (UKPDS 33). *Lancet* 1998; 352: 837–853.
2.   UK Prospective Diabetes Study Group. Tight blood pressure control and risk of macrovascular and microvascular complications in type 2 diabetes (UKPDS 38). *BMJ* 1998; 317: 703–713.

B.   Diabetic Control and Complication Trial (DCCT)

Aim of study: The role of intensive glycemic control on diabetic retinopathy in Type 1 DM .

Study Design: Randomized controlled trial.

Results: The DCCT randomized 1441 patients with type 1 diabetes to receive intensive glycaemic or conventional therapy. Over 6.5 years of follow-up, intensive treatment (median HbA1c, 7.2%) reduced the incidence of diabetic retinopathy by 76% and the progression of diabetic retinopathy by 54%, as compared with the conventional treatment. On the long-term, the rate of progression of retinopathy is slower in the tight control group. Early worsening of diabetic retinopathy was noticed in the tight control group. However, the long-term benefit was significant. Laser treatment is advised early in the patients with high risk retinopathy before putting them on intensive treatment.

Importance of study: The DCCT showed that tight control in Type 1 Diabetes can reduce retinopathy and slow down the progression.

Reference
1.   The Diabetes Control and Complications Trial Research Group. The effect of intensive treatment of diabetes on the development and progression of long- term complications in insulin-dependent diabetes mellitus. *N Engl J Med* 1993; 329: 977–986.

C.   Diabetic Retinopathy Study (DRS)
Aim: To determine the role of PRP in reducing VA loss in advanced DR.

Design: Multi-centre, randomized trial: argon or xenon PRP versus no treatment.

Methodology: The patients' eyes were randomized to receive either laser photocoagulation or follow-up with no treatment. The photocoagulation was either by xenon or argon by randomization. Best corrected visual acuity was assessed every 4 months.

Results
1..   Primary Outcome
Visual acuity: Severe visual loss (VA <5/200) was reduced by either methods by 50% .
2.   Secondary Outcomes
Progression of retinopathy: Scatter photocoagulation with both argon and xenon reduced the rate of progression of eyes to more severe stages of proliferative diabetic retinopathy compared with no treatment.
IOP: Panretinal photocoagulation reduced the risk of elevated intraocular pressure, possibly preventing the development of neovascular glaucoma.

Risk Factors: Four risk factors were identified for increasing the risk of severe visual acuity loss in untreated eyes:
- presence of vitreous or preretinal haemorrages
- presence of new vessels
- location of new vessels on or near the disc
- severity of new vessels

Of these, neovascularisation of the disc had the strongest association with severe visual acuity loss among untreated eyes. Presence of any of these risk factors was considered an indicator for treatment with PRP.

Risks of treatment: PRP was associated with mild loss of vision soon after treatment, particularly in eyes with pre-existing macular oedema. However, long-term benefits outweighed the risk of visual loss.

Importance of study: The DRS was a seminal clinical trial, as it provided a firm evidence-base for the effectiveness of PRP in reducing the progression of proliferative diabetic retinopathy and severe sight loss in high-risk diabetic retinopathy eyes.

References:

1.   Diabetic Retinopathy Study Research Group. Preliminary report on effects of photocoagulation therapy. *Am J Ophthalmology* 1976; 81: 383-396.

2.   Diabetic Retinopathy Study Research Group. Photocoagulation treatment of proliferative diabetic retinopathy: The second report of Diabetic Retinopathy Study findings. *Ophthalmology* 1978; 85: 82-106.

D.   Early Treatment Diabetic Retinopathy Study (ETDRS)

Aim: The efficacy of argon laser photocoagulation and aspirin in diabetic retinopathy.

Design: Multi-centre, randomized controlled trial.

Methods: All patients were assigned to either aspirin treatment or placebo during the course of the study. Additionally, one eye of each patient was assigned to immediate laser. Two types of laser were analyzed in the study: focal macular laser and peripheral scatter laser. Eyes selected for immediate treatment received one of four different combinations of focal and scatter treatment. By varying the amount of scatter treatment given and the time of initiation of focal treatment for macular oedema, the study investigators hoped to find the best possible early treatment strategy.

Results

1.   *Aspirin*

Aspirin use did not affect the progression of retinopathy to the high-risk proliferative stage in eyes assigned to deferral of photocoagulation. However, aspirin did not increase the risk of vitreous haemorrhage, did not affect vision, and was associated with a decreased risk of cardiovascular disease.

2.   *Focal macular laser*

The ETDRS demonstrated that focal macular laser reduced the risk of moderate vision loss (defined as a doubling of the visual angle) by up to 50% in eyes with 'clinically significant macular oedema'. There was also an increase of moderate visual gain in eyes receiving focal treatment as well as a decrease in the amount of retinal thickening. The recommendation was that eyes with clinically significant macular oedema should be considered for focal photocoagulation.

3.   *Scatter PRP*

The ETDRS study demonstrated a statistically significant reduction in severe visual loss in eyes receiving early scatter laser treatment, especially for those patients with non-insulin-dependent diabetes mellitus (NIDDM). The recommendation was that scatter treatment should be deferred for eyes with mild to moderate non-proliferative diabetic retinopathy. As the retinopathy progresses to the severe non-proliferative or early proliferative stage, scatter treatment should be considered, especially for patients with NIDDM. Scatter photocoagulation should be performed for virtually all eyes with high-risk proliferative retinopathy. Finally, early vitrectomy should be considered for advanced active proliferative diabetic retinopathy and, most importantly, all patients with diabetic retinopathy should receive careful follow-up.

Importance of study: The ETDRS study was a landmark trial in that it demonstrated conclusively the benefit of focal macular laser in the treatment of diabetic macular oedema and scatter laser PRP for severe NPDR and PDR. It also concluded that aspirin intake did not affect the progression of retinopathy.

References

1.   Fong DS, Ferris FL, Davis MD, Chew EY, ETDRS Research Group. Causes of severe visual loss in the Early Treatment Diabetic Retinopathy Study. ETDRS Report No. 24. *Am J Ophthalmol* 1999; 127: 137-141.

2.   Fong DS, Barton FB, Bresnick GH, ETDRS Research Group. Impaired color vision associated with diabetic retinopathy: Early Treatment Diabetic Retinopathy Study. ETDRS Report No. 15. *Am J Ophthalmol* 1999; 128: 612-617.

3.   Chew EY, Klein ML, Ferris FL III, Remaley NA, Murphy RP, Chantry K, Hoogwerf BJ, Miller D, Early Treatment Diabetic Retinopathy Study Research Group. Association of elevated serum lipid levels with retinal hard exudate in diabetic retinopathy. ETDRS Report Number 22. *Arch Ophthalmol* 1996; 114: 1079-1084.

4.   Ferris FL. Early photocoagulation in patients with either type 1 or type II diabetes. *Tr Am Ophth Soc* 1996; 94: 505-537.

5.   Ferris FL, Chew EY, Hoogwerf BJ, Early Treatment Diabetic Retinopathy Study Research Group: Serum lipids and diabetic retinopathy. *Diabetes Care* 1996; 19: 1291-1293.

6.   Braun CI, Benson WE, Remaley NA, Chew EY, Ferris FL, Early Treatment Diabetic Retinopathy Study Research Group. Accommodation amplitudes in the Early Treatment Diabetic Retinopathy Study. ETDRS Report Number 21. *Retina* 1995; 15: 275-281.

7.   Chew EY, Klein ML, Murphy RP, Remaley NA, Ferris FL, Early Treatment Diabetic Retinopathy Study Research Group. Effects of aspirin on preretinal hemorrhage in patients with diabetes mellitus. ETDRS Report Number 20. *Arch Ophthalmol* 1995; 113: 52-55.

8.   Early Treatment Diabetic Retinopathy Study Research Group. Focal photocoagulation treatment of diabetic macular edema. ETDRS Report Number 19. *Arch Ophthalmol* 1995; 113: 1144-1155.

9.   Ferris FL. How effective are treatments for diabetic retinopathy? (commentary). *JAMA* 1993; 269: 1290-1291.

10.   Prior MJ, Prout T, Miller D, Ewart R, Kumar D, Early Treatment Diabetic Retinopathy Research Group. C-peptide and the classification of diabetes patients in the Early Treatment Diabetic Retinopathy Study. ETDRS Report Number 6. *Ann Epidemiol* 1993; 3: 9-17, 1993.

11.   Early Treatment Diabetic Retinopathy Study Investigators. Aspirin effects on mortality and morbidity in patients with diabetes mellitus. ETDRS Report 14. *JAMA* 1992; 268: 1292-1300.

12.   Chew EY, Williams GA, Burton TC, Barton FB, Remaley NA, Ferris FL, Early Treatment Diabetic Retinopathy Study Research Group. Aspirin effects on the development of cataracts in patients with diabetes mellitus. ETDRS Report Number 16. *Arch Ophthalmol* 1992; 110: 339-342.

13. Flynn HW, Chew EY, Simmons BD, Barton FB, Remaley NA, Ferris FL, Early Treatment Diabetic Retinopathy Study Research Group. Pars Plana Vitrectomy in the Early Treatment Diabetic Retinopathy Study. ETDRS Report Number 17. *Ophthalmology* 1992; 99: 1351-1357.

14. Early Treatment Diabetic Retinopathy Study Research Group. Early Treatment Diabetic Retinopathy Study design and baseline patient characteristics. ETDRS Report Number 7. *Ophthalmology* 1991; 98: 741-756.

15. Early Treatment Diabetic Retinopathy Study Research Group. Effects of aspirin treatment on diabetic retinopathy. ETDRS Report Number 8. *Ophthalmology* 1991; 98: 757-765.

16. Early Treatment Diabetic Retinopathy Study Research Group. Early photocoagulation for diabetic retinopathy. ETDRS Report Number 9. *Ophthalmology* 1991; 98: 766-785.

17. Early Treatment Diabetic Retinopathy Study Research Group. Grading diabetic retinopathy from stereoscopic color fundus photographs: An extension of the modified Airlie House classification. ETDRS Report Number 10. *Ophthalmology* 1991; 98: 786-806.

18. Early Treatment Diabetic Retinopathy Study Research Group. Classification of diabetic retinopathy from fluorescein angiograms. ETDRS Report Number 11. *Ophthalmology* 1991; 98: 807-822.

19. Early Treatment Diabetic Retinopathy Study Research Group. Fundus photographic risk factors for progression of diabetic retinopathy. ETDRS Report Number 12. *Ophthalmology* 1991; 98: 823-833.

20. Early Treatment Diabetic Retinopathy Study Research Group. Fluorescein angiographic risk factors for progression of diabetic retinopathy. ETDRS Report Number 13. *Ophthalmology* 1991; 98: 834-840.

21. Kinyoun J, Barton F, Fisher M, Hubbard LL, Aiello L, Ferris FL, Early Treatment Diabetic Retinopathy Study Research Group. Detection of diabetic macular edema. Ophthalmoscopy versus photography. ETDRS Report Number 5. *Ophthalmology* 1989; 69: 746-751.

22. Early Treatment Diabetic Retinopathy Study Research Group. Treatment techniques and clinical guidelines for photocoagulation of diabetic macular edema. Early Treatment Diabetic Retinopathy Study Report Number 2. *Ophthalmology* 1987; 94: 761-774.

23. Early Treatment Diabetic Retinopathy Study Research Group. Techniques for scatter and local photocoagulation treatment of diabetic retinopathy. Early Treatment Diabetic Retinopathy Study Report Number 3. *Int Ophthalmol Clin* 19878; 27: 254-264.

24. Early Treatment Diabetic Retinopathy Study Research Group. Photocoagulation for diabetic macular edema. Early Treatment Diabetic Retinopathy Study Report Number 4. Int Ophthalmol Clin 1987; 27: 265-272.

25. Photocoagulation for diabetic macular edema. Early Treatment Diabetic Retinopathy Study Report Number 1. *Arch Ophthalmol* 1985; 103: 1796.

E.   Diabetic Vitrectomy Study

Aim: Early versus deferred vitrectomy following vitreous haemorrhage.

Design: Randomized controlled trial.

Methodology: The Diabetic Retinopathy Vitrectomy Study (DRVS) randomized 616 eyes with recent vitreous haemorrhage, reducing visual acuity to 5/200 or less for at least 1 month to undergo early vitrectomy within 6 months or deferral of vitrectomy for 1 year. After 2 years of follow-up, 25% of the patients in the early vitrectomy group had visual acuity of 10/20 or better compared with 15% in the deferral group. In patients with type 1 diabetes, who were on average younger and had more severe PDR, there was a clear-cut advantage for early vitrectomy, as reflected in the percentage of eyes recovering visual acuity of 10/20 or better (36% versus 12% in the deferral group). No such advantage was found in the type 2 diabetes group (16% in the early group versus 18% in the deferral group).

Reference

1.   The Diabetic Retinopathy Vitrectomy Study Research Group. Early vitrectomy for severe vitreous hemorrhage in diabetic retinopathy. Two-year results of a randomized trial. *Arch Ophthalmol* 1985; 103:1644–1652.

F.   DRCRNET Study for DME

Aim: Randomized trial evaluating ranibizumab plus prompt or deferred laser or triamcinolone plus prompt laser for diabetic macular oedema. Evaluate intravitreal 0.5 mg ranibizumab or 4mg triamcinolone combined with focal/grid laser compared with focal/grid laser alone for the treatment of diabetic macular oedema (DME).

Design: Multi-centre, randomized clinical trial.

Participants: A total of 854 eyes of 691 participants with visual acuity (approximate Snellen equivalent) of 20/32 to 20/320 and DME involving the fovea.

Methods: Eyes were randomized to sham injection + prompt laser (n=293), 0.5 mg ranibizumab + prompt laser (n=187), 0.5 mg ranibizumab + deferred (≥24 weeks) laser (n=188), or 4 mg triamcinolone + prompt laser (n=186). Retreatment followed an algorithm facilitated by a web-based, real-time data-entry system.

Main outcome measures: Best-corrected visual acuity and safety at 1 year.

Results: The 1-year mean change (±standard deviation) in the visual acuity letter score from baseline was significantly greater in the ranibizumab + prompt laser group (+9±11, P<0.001) and the ranibizumab + deferred laser group (+9±12, P<0.001), but not in the triamcinolone + prompt laser group (+4±13, P=0.31), compared with the sham + prompt laser group (+3±13). Reduction in the mean central subfield thickness in the triamcinolone + prompt laser group was similar to both ranibizumab groups and greater than in the sham + prompt laser group. In the subset of pseudophakic eyes at baseline (n=273), visual acuity improvement in the triamcinolone +prompt laser group appeared comparable to that in the ranibizumab groups. No systemic events attributable to the study treatment were apparent. Three eyes (0.8%) had injection-related endophthalmitis in the ranibizumab groups, while elevated intraocular pressure and cataract surgery were more frequent in the triamcinolone + prompt laser group. Two-year visual acuity outcomes were similar to 1-year outcomes.

Conclusions: Intravitreal ranibizumab with prompt or deferred laser is more effective through at least 1 year compared with prompt laser alone for the treatment of DME involving the central macula. Ranibizumab, as applied in this study, although uncommonly associated with endophthalmitis, should be considered for patients with DME and characteristics similar to those in this clinical trial. In pseudophakic eyes, intravitreal triamcinolone + prompt laser seems more effective than laser alone, but frequently increases the risk of intraocular pressure elevation.

Reference

1.   DRCR.net, Elman MJ, Aiello LP, Beck RW, Bressler NM, Bressler SB, Edwards AR, et al. Randomized trial evaluating ranibizumab plus prompt or deferred laser or triamcinolone plus prompt laser for diabetic macular edema. *Ophthalmology* 2010; 117(6): 1064–1077.

G.   DCRNET STUDY- Laser vs Ranibizumab for PDR

Aim: Panretinal photocoagulation vs intravitreous ranibizumab for proliferative diabetic retinopathy.

Design: Randomized trial

Importance: Panretinal photocoagulation (PRP) is the standard treatment for reducing severe visual loss from proliferative diabetic retinopathy. However, PRP can damage the retina, resulting in peripheral vision loss or worsening diabetic macular oedema (DME).

Objective: To evaluate the noninferiority of intravitreous ranibizumab compared with PRP for visual acuity outcomes in patients with proliferative diabetic retinopathy.

Design, setting and participants: Randomized clinical trial conducted at 55 US sites among 305 adults with proliferative diabetic retinopathy enrolled between February and December 2012 (mean age, 52 years; 44% female; 52% white). Both eyes were enrolled for 89 participants (1 eye to each study group), with a total of 394 eyes. The final 2-year visit was completed in January 2015.

Interventions: Individual eyes were randomly assigned to receive PRP treatment, completed in 1 to 3 visits (n = 203 eyes) or ranibizumab, 0.5 mg by intravitreous injection at baseline and as frequently as every 4 weeks based on a structured re-treatment protocol (n = 191 eyes). Eyes in both treatment groups could receive ranibizumab for DME.

Main outcomes and measures: The primary outcome was mean visual acuity change at 2 years (5-letter noninferiority margin; intention to-treat analysis). Secondary outcomes included visual acuity area under the curve, peripheral visual field loss, vitrectomy, DME development and retinal neovascularization.

Results: Mean visual acuity letter improvement at 2 years was +2.8 in the ranibizumab group vs +0.2 in the PRP group (difference, +2.2; 95% CI, –0.5 to +5.0; P < .001 for noninferiority). The mean treatment group difference in visual acuity area under the curve over 2 years was +4.2 (95% CI, +3.0 to +5.4; P < .001). Mean peripheral visual field sensitivity loss was worse (–23 dB vs –422 dB; difference, 372 dB; 95% CI, 213-531 dB;P < .001), vitrectomy was more frequent (15% vs 4%; difference, 9%; 95% CI, 4%-15%; P < .001), and DME development was more frequent (28% vs 9%; difference, 19%;

95% CI, 10%-28%; P < .001) in the PRP group vs differences between groups in rates of major cardiovascular events were identified.

Conclusions and relevance: Among eyes with proliferative diabetic retinopathy, treatment with ranibizumab resulted in visual acuity that was noninferior to (not worse than) PRP treatment at 2 years. Although longer-term follow-up is needed, ranibizumab may be a reasonable treatment alternative, at least through 2 years for patients with proliferative diabetic retinopathy.

Reference
1.   Diabetic Retinopathy Clinical Research Network. Panretinal photocoagulation vs intravitreous ranibizumab for proliferative diabetic retinopathy: A randomized trial. *JAMA* 2015; 314(20): 2137-2146.

H.   DCRNET STUDY- Aflibercept, Bevacizumab and Ranibizumab for DME
Aim: Compare aflibercept, bevacizumab or ranibizumab for diabetic macular oedema.

Design: Randomized trial.

Method: At 89 clinical sites, 660 adults (mean age, 61±10 years) with diabetic macular oedema involving the macular centre received intravitreous aflibercept at a dose of 2.0 mg (224 participants), bevacizumab at a dose of 1.25 mg (218 participants) and ranibizumab at a dose of 0.3 mg (218 participants). The study drugs were administered as often as every 4 weeks, according to a protocol-specified algorithm. The primary outcome was the mean change in visual acuity at 1 year.

Results: From baseline to 1 year, the mean visual acuity letter score (range, 0 to 100, with higher scores indicating better visual acuity; a score of 85 is approximately 20/20) improved by 13.3 with aflibercept, by 9.7 with bevacizumab, and by 11.2 with ranibizumab. Although the improvement was greater with aflibercept than with the other two drugs (P<0.001 for aflibercept vs. bevacizumab and P = 0.03 for aflibercept vs. ranibizumab), it was not clinically meaningful, because the difference was driven by the eyes with worse visual acuity at baseline (P<0.001 for interaction). When the initial visual acuity letter score was 78 to 69 (equivalent to approximately 20/32 to 20/40) (51% of participants), the mean improvement was 8.0 with aflibercept, 7.5 with bevacizumab, and 8.3 with ranibizumab (P>0.50 for each pairwise comparison). When the initial letter score was less than 69 (approximately 20/50 or worse), the mean improvement was 18.9 with aflibercept, 11.8 with bevacizumab and 14.2 with ranibizumab (P<0.001 for aflibercept vs. bevacizumab, P = 0.003 for aflibercept vs. ranibizumab, and P = 0.21 for ranibizumab vs. bevacizumab). There was no significant difference between the study groups in the rates of serious adverse events (P = 0.40), hospitalization (P = 0.51), death (P = 0.72) or major cardiovascular events (P = 0.56).

Conclusion: Intravitreous aflibercept, bevacizumab or ranibizumab improved vision in eyes with centre-involved diabetic macular oedema, but the relative effect depended on baseline visual acuity. When the initial visual acuity loss was mild, there was no apparent difference between the study groups. At worse levels of initial visual acuity, aflibercept was more effective at improving vision.

Reference

1. Diabetic Retinopathy Clinical Research Network, Wells JA, Glassman AR, Ayala AR, Jampol LM, Aiello LP, Antoszyk AN, Arnold-Bush B, Baker CW, Bressler NM, Browning DJ, Elman MJ, Ferris FL, Friedman SM, Melia M, Pieramici DJ, Sun JK, Beck RW. Aflibercept, bevacizumab, or ranibizumab for diabetic macular edema. N Engl J Med. 2015 Mar 26; 372(13): 1193–1203.

I. Age-Related Eye Disease Study

Aim: Efficacy of vitamin and mineral supplements in preventing AMD and cataract.

Design: Multi-centre, randomized, double masked, placebo-controlled trial.

Methods: The antioxidant formulation contained a combination of vitamin C, vitamin E and beta-carotene. The specific daily amounts of antioxidants and zinc used by the AREDS researchers were:

- 500 milligrams of vitamin C
- 400 international units of vitamin E
- 15 milligrams of beta-carotene
- 80 milligrams of zinc as zinc oxide
- 2 milligrams of copper as cupric oxide

Results: Antioxidants plus zinc reduced the risk of developing advanced AMD by about 25% and reduced risk of vision loss by about 19%. Zinc alone reduced the risk of developing advanced AMD by about 21% and reduced risk of vision loss by about 11%. Antioxidants alone reduced the risk of developing advanced AMD by about 17% and reduced the risk of vision loss by about 10%.

Recommendations: Early dry AMD with a few small/medium drusens, normal vision requires no treatment. Intermediate and advanced AMD, especially involving one eye, require supplements. The study found that there was no protective effect and therefore supplements have no role in cataract prevention.

Reference

1. A randomized, placebo controlled, clinical trial of high-dose supplementation with vitamins C and E, beta carotene, and zinc for age-related macular degeneration and vision loss: AREDS report no. 8. *Ophthalmol.* 2001; 119(10): 1417-36.

2. A randomized, placebo-controlled, clinical trial of high-dose supplementation with vitamins C and E and beta carotene for age related cataract and vision loss: AREDS report no. 9. *Arch Ophthalmol.* 2001; 119(10): 1439-52.

J.   AREDS 2 STUDY – The Age-Related Eye Disease Study 2 (AREDS2) Randomized Clinical Trial

Aim: To determine whether adding lutein + zeaxanthin, DHA + EPA or both to the AREDS formulation decreases the risk of developing advanced AMD. To evaluate the effect of eliminating beta carotene, lowering zinc doses or both in the AREDS formulation.

Methodology: Participants were randomized to receive lutein (10 mg) + zeaxanthin (2 mg), DHA (350 mg) + EPA (650 mg), lutein + zeaxanthin and DHA + EPA or placebo. All participants were also asked to take the original AREDS formulation or accept a secondary randomization to 4 variations of the AREDS formulation, including elimination of beta carotene, lowering of zinc dose or both.

Main outcomes and measures: Development of advanced AMD. The unit of analyses used was by eye.

Results: Median follow-up was 5 years, with 1940 study eyes (1608 participants) progressing to advanced AMD. Kaplan-Meier probabilities of progression to advanced AMD by 5 years were 31% (493 eyes [406 participants]) for placebo, 29% (468 eyes [399 participants]) for lutein + zeaxanthin, 31% (507 eyes [416 participants]) for DHA + EPA, and 30% (472 eyes [387 participants]) for lutein + zeaxanthin and DHA + EPA. There was no apparent effect of beta carotene elimination or lower-dose zinc on progression to advanced AMD. More lung cancers were noted in the beta carotene vs no beta carotene group (23 [2.0%] vs 11 [0.9%], nominal P = .04), mostly in former smokers.

Conclusions and relevance: Addition of lutein + zeaxanthin, DHA + EPA or both to the AREDS formulation in primary analyses did not further reduce the risk of progression to advanced AMD. However, because of potential increased incidence of lung cancer in former smokers, lutein + zeaxanthin could be an appropriate carotenoid substitute in the AREDS formulation.

Reference

1.   The Age-Related Eye Disease Study 2 (AREDS2) Research Group. Acids for age-related macular degeneration: The Age-Related Eye Disease Study 2 (AREDS2) Randomized Clinical Trial. *JAMA* 2013; 309(19): 2005-2015.

K.   ANCHOR Trial

Aim: Safety and efficacy of monthly ranibizumab vs PDT in classic wet AMD.

Design: Multi-centre, randomized, double blind clinical trial.

Methodology: The ANCHOR trial recruited 423 patients with predominantly classic CNVM across multiple centres in the United States, Europe and Australia (visual acuity between 6/12 and 6/90). Patients were randomized in a 1:1:1 ratio between (1) monthly ranibizumab 0.3mg plus sham PDT, or (2) monthly ranibizumab 0.5mg plus sham PDT, or (3) standard protocol PDT plus monthly sham injections. Fluoroscein angiography was performed every 3 months in all patients to determine the need for additional PDT or sham PDT. Primary efficacy endpoint was pre-specified as the proportion of patients losing fewer than 15 letters between baseline and 12 months.

Results: Patients losing fewer than 15 letters at 12 months: 96% Ranibizumab 0.5mg, 94% ranibizumab 0.3mg, 64% PDT (p<0.0001). Patients gaining 15 letters or more at 12 months: 40% ranibizumab 0.5mg, 36% ranibizumab 0.3mg, 6% PDT (p< 0.0001). Average letters gained or lost: 11 letters gained. Ranibizumab 0.5mg: 9 letters gained. Ranibizumab 0.3mg: 10 letters lost PDT (p<0.0001). Severe vision loss: 0% Ranibizumab, 13% PDT.

Adverse events
- Endophthalmitis: 0% (0.3mg Ranibizumab) and 1.4% (0.5mg Ranibizumab)
- Uveitis: 10.2% (0.3mg Ranibizumab), 15% (0.5mg Ranibizumab) and 2.8% (PDT)
- Non-ocular vascular events: 2.2% (0.3g Ranibizumab) and 4.3% (0.5mg Ranibizumab) and 2.1% (PDT)

Conclusion: Ranibizumab is superior and produced visual acuity gain, while PDT produced visual acuity loss.

Reference
1.   Brown DM, Brown DM1, Kaiser PK, Michels M, Soubrane G, Heier JS, et al. Ranibizumab versus verteporfin for neovascular age-related macular degeneration. *N Engl J Med*. 2006; 355(14): 1432-44.

L.   MARINA Study

Aim: Efficacy of monthly ranibizumab for treating minimally classic and occult CNVM.

Design: Multi-centre, randomized, double blind sham-controlled.

Method: 716 patients (VA 6/12 to 6/96) were randomized to receive monthly intravitreal injections of ranibizumab (either 0.3mg or 0.5mg) or sham injections for 24 months. The primary endpoint was the proportion of patients losing fewer than 15 letters from baseline acuity at 12 months.

Results: Patients losing fewer than 15 letters at 12 months: 95% treatment groups vs 62% in the sham group (p<0.0001). Patients gaining more than 15 letters at 12 months: 25% and 34% treated groups (0.3mg and 0.5mg, respectively) vs 5% controls. Average change in visual acuity: 7 letters gained in the treated groups vs 10 letters lost in the controls.

Adverse events: Endophthalmitis (<1%), uveitis (<1%) and serious non-ocular events were not significantly different in the treated groups vs control group.

M.   CATT Trial

Aim: To determine the relative efficacy and safety of ranibizumab versus bevacizumab for the treatment of wet AMD. To determine the relative efficacy and safety of monthly versus PRN dosing for each drug.

Design: Multi-centre, randomized controlled trial.

Results:

Ranibizumab versus Bevacizuamab

- 1 year: Ranibizumab and bevacizumab had equivalent effects on visual acuity at all time points throughout the first year of follow-up, including the mean number of letters gained, the proportion of patients in whom visual acuity was maintained by less than 15 letters, and the proportion who gained greater than 15 letters, when comparing the same dosing regimens.
- 2 years: Most of the change in VA occurred in the first year. At 2 years, there was no statistically significant difference in VA outcomes between ranibizumab and bevacizumab when comparing either monthly or PRN groups.

Monthly versus PRN Regimes

- 1 year: Ranibizumab given as needed was equivalent to ranibizumab given monthly, with a mean difference of 1.7 letters. Bevacizumab given as needed was equivalent to bevacizumab given monthly at all time points through 36 weeks (with mean difference all within 1.6 letters); at 52 weeks, the difference of 2.1 letters yielded an inconclusive comparison.
- 2 years: After adjusting for predictors in a multi-variate model, patients treated monthly for 2 years performed 1.7 letters better than patients treated PRN for 2 years. But this was not statistically significant at the 5% level.

Switching from monthly to PRN at 1 year

Switching to as-needed dosing after 1 year of monthly treatment, with either drug, produced a mean 2.2-letter decrease compared to those treated monthly throughout 2 years and yielded a mean visual acuity nearly equal to that obtained with as-needed dosing throughout 2 years.

Side effects

- *1 year*: No significant differences between the two drugs in rates of death, arteriothrombotic events, or venous thrombotic events were found. However, the rate of serious systemic adverse events, primarily hospitalizations, was higher among bevacizumab-treated patients than among ranibizumab-treated patients (24.1% vs. 19.0%, P=0.04).
- *2 years*: Again, there was no diference in rates of death or arteriothrombotic events such as MI and stroke between ranibizumab and bevacizumab. However, the higher rate of serious systemic effects (including hospitalizations) noted at 1 year continued through year 2. The greatest imbalance was in gastrointestinal disorders. When known adverse events of anti-VEGF were excluded from the analysis, most of the imbalance remained making it unsure if this difference occurred by chance, due to imbalances at baseline not captured in multivariate modeling, or truly a higher risk.

Importance of the CATT Trial: The CATT trial provided evidence that bevacizumab is an effective alternative to ranibizumab in the treatment of wet AMD at the 1-year and 2-year time-points. Visual acuity outcomes were not statistically different between the drugs, when the same dosing regimens were compared. Also, the trial confirmed that as required dosing is an effective means of administration of both anti-VEGF agents, and was not proven to be inferior to monthly dosing for either drug.

References

1. CATT Research Group, Martin DF, Maguire MG, Ying GS, Grunwald JE, Fine SL, Jaffe GJ. Ranibizumab and bevacizumab for neovascular age-related macular degeneration. *N Engl J Med* 2011; 364(20): 1897-1908.
2. Comparison of Age-related Macular Degeneration Treatments Trials (CATT) Research Group, Martin DF, Maguire MG, et al. Ranibizumab and bevacizumab for treatment of neovascular age-related macular degeneration: two-year results. *Ophthalmology* 2012; 119(7):1388-98.

N.   The Branch Vein Occlusion Study (BRVO Study)

Aim: Role of grid laser for CMO and PRP for neovascularization in BRVO.

Design: Multi-centre, randomized, controlled clinical trial.

Results

Outcome 1: Efficacy of Macular Grid Laser
- 139 eyes included in study with a mean follow-up of 3 years.
- The gain of at least two lines of visual acuity from baseline maintained for two consecutive visits was significantly greater in treated eyes (P = .00049, logrank test).

The results of the BVOS trial established macular grid laser as the gold standard treatment for macular oedema due to branch retinal vein occlusions for the better part of 2 decades. Recent evidence suggests that newer treatment modalities such as intra-vitreal steroids and anti-VEGF agents - may be more efficacious than laser in this condition.

Outcome 2 - Efficacy of Sectoral PRP
In the 319 eyes without neovascularisation, treated eyes developed significantly less neovascularisation (P<0.009) than non-treated eyes over the course of follow-up (mean follow-up of 3.7 years). In the 82 eyes with neovascularisation, treated eyes developed significantly less vitreous haemorrhage (P=0.005). This study established sectoral scatter PRP as the gold-standard for the prevention of neovascularisation and vitreous haemorrhage in branch vein occlusions. Though not a specified outcome of the study, the authors recommend that sectoral PRP should be performed once neovascularisation is detected and need not be performed prophylactically.

References

1. The Branch Vein Occlusion Study Group. Argon laser photocoagulation for macular edema in branch vein occlusion. *Am J Ophthalmol.* 1984; 98(3): 271-282.

2.   The Branch Vein Occlusion Study Group. Argon laser scatter photocoagulation for prevention of neovascularization and vitreous hemorrhage in branch vein occlusion. A randomized clinical trial. *Arch Ophthalmology* 1986 104; 34-41.

O.   The Central Retinal Vein Occlusion Study (CRVO Study)

Aim: Role of macular grid laser for treating CMO secondary to CRVO.

Design: Multi-centre, randomizsed, controlled clinical trial.

Methods:
Eyes were assigned to either macular grid photocoagulation or no treatment and follow-up was every 4 months for 3 years.

Inclusion criteria
*   Angiographically documented macular oedema secondary to CRVO.
*   Best-corrected visual acuity of 20/50 or worse.

Primary outcome: The main outcome measure was visual acuity.

Results: There was no statistically significant difference between treatment and control visual acuity at any stage of follow-up. Initial visual acuity: 20/160 (treated) vs. 20/125 (control). Final visual acuity: 20/200 (treated) vs. 20/160 (control).

Conclusions: The results of the study did not support a recommendation for macular grid laser for CRVO. PRP is beneficial only when NVI or NVG develops.

Reference
1.   The Central Vein Occlusion Study Group. Evaluation of grid pattern photocoagulation for macular edema in central vein occlusion. The Central Vein Occlusion Study Group M report. *Ophthalmology* 1995; 102(10): 1425-1433.

P.   BRAVO Study

Aim: Efficacy and safety of ranibizumab injection compared with sham in patients with macular oedema secondary to BRVO.

Design: A phase 3, multicentre, randomized, sham injection-controlled study.

Methodology: Patients were randomly assigned to 6 monthly injections of ranibizumab, either 0.3 mg or 0.5 mg, or to sham injections. The primary efficacy outcome was mean change from baseline BCVA at 6 months. Secondary outcomes include the percentage of patients who gained 3 lines (15 letters) of BCVA at 6 months. Patients were eligible for laser rescue treatment at 3 months if macular oedema showed little or no improvement, visual acuity was 20/40 or worse, and central subfield thickness was 250 μm or greater.

Inclusion criteria: Patients included in the study had macular oedema involving the foveal centre secondary to BRVO, central subfield macular thickness of 250 μm or greater on optical coherence tomography, and BCVA of 20/40 to 20/400.

Results: In 397 patients randomized, the mean gain from baseline at month 6 was 16.6 letters in patients receiving 0.3 mg of ranibizumab, 18.3 letters in those receiving 0.5 mg, and 7.3 in those receiving sham injection. Improvement in BCVA was evident as early as 1 week, with patients achieving a mean gain of 7.6, 7.4, and 1.9 letters in the 0.3 mg and 0.5 mg ranibizumab and sham groups at 1 week, respectively. By month 6, most patients in the two ranibizumab groups gained at least 3 lines of BCVA (55.2% in the 0.3 mg group and 61.1% in the 0.5 mg group), while most of those in the sham group did not (28.8%).

Reference

1.   Campochiaro PA, Heier JS, Feiner L, Gray S, Saroj N, Rundle AC, Murahashi WY, Rubio RG, BRAVO Investigators. Ranibizumab for macular edema following branch retinal vein occlusion: Six-month primary end point results of a phase III study. *Ophthalmology* 2010; 117(6):1102-1112..

Q.   CRUISE Study

Aim: Efficacy and safety of ranibizumab injection compared with sham in patients with macular oedema secondary to CRVO. To assess the efficacy and safety of ranibizumab injection compared with sham in patients with macular oedema secondary to CRVO.

Design: A phase 3, multicentre, randomized, sham injection-controlled study.

Methodology: Patients were randomly assigned to 6 monthly intravitreal injections of 0.3mg or 0.5mg ranibizumab or sham injection. The primary efficacy outcome was mean change from baseline BCVA at 6 months. Secondary outcomes included the percentage of patients who gained 3 lines (15 letters) of BCVA at 6 months.

Inclusion criteria: Macular oedema involving the foveal centre secondary to CRVO, central subfield macular thickness of 250 μm or greater on optical coherence tomography and BCVA of 20/40 to 20/320.

Results: In 392 randomized patients, the mean gain from baseline BCVA at month 6 was 12.7 letters in patients who received 0.3 mg ranibizumab, 14.9 letters in patients who received 0.5mg ranibizumab, and 0.8 letters in those who received sham injections. Again, gain in BCVA was seen as early as 1 week, with patients achieving mean gains of 8.8, 9.3, and 1.1 letters in the 0.3mg and 0.5 mg ranibizumab and sham groups at 1 week. At month 6, gains of three lines or more in BCVA were seen in 46.2% of patients receiving 0.3 mg ranibizumab, 47.7 of those receiving 0.5 mg ranibizumab, and 16.9% of those receiving sham injections.

References

1.   Brown DM, Campochiaro PA, Singh RP, et al. *Ophthalmology* 2010; 117(6): 1124 –1133.

R.   Endophthalmitis Vitrectomy Study

Aim: To determine the role of immediate pars plana vitrectomy (VIT) and systemic antibiotic treatment in the management of postoperative endophthalmitis.

Design: Investigator-initiated, multicentre, randomized clinical trial.

Methodology: A total of 420 patients who had clinical evidence of endophthalmitis within 6 weeks after cataract surgery or secondary intraocular lens implantation.

Interventions: Random assignment according to a 2 x 2 factorial design to treatment with VIT or vitreous tap or biopsy (TAP) and to treatment with or without systemic antibiotics (ceftazidime and amikacin).

Main Outcome Measures: A 9-month evaluation of visual acuity assessed by an Early Treatment Diabetic Retinopathy Study acuity chart and media clarity assessed both clinically and photographically.

Results: There was no difference in final visual acuity or media clarity with or without the use of systemic antibiotics. In patients whose initial visual acuity was hand motions or better, there was no difference in visual outcome whether or not an immediate VIT was performed. However, in the subgroup of patients with initial light perception-only vision, VIT produced a threefold increase in the frequency of achieving 20/40 or better acuity (33% vs 11%), approximately a twofold chance of achieving 20/100 or better acuity (56% vs 30%), and a 50% decrease in the frequency of severe visual loss (20% vs 47%) over TAP. In this group of patients, the difference between VIT and TAP was statistically significant ($P < .001$, logrank test for cumulative visual acuity scores) over the entire range of vision.

Conclusions: Omission of systemic antibiotic treatment can reduce toxic effects, costs and length of hospital stay. Routine immediate VIT is not necessary in patients with better than light perception vision at presentation, but is of substantial benefit for those who have light perception-only vision.

Reference:

1.   Endophthalmitis Vitrectomy Study Group. Results of the Endophthalmitis Vitrectomy Study. A randomized trial of immediate vitrectomy and of intravenous antibiotics for the treatment of postoperative bacterial endophthalmitis. *Arch Ophthalmol.* 1995;113(12): 1479-96.

Retinal Studies from the Author

1.   **Oluleye TS, Ajaiyeoba AI. Retinal diseases in Ibadan.** *Eye* **2006; 20(12): 1461-3.**
Aim: To determine the common retinal diseases in Ibadan with a view to set up a vitreo-retinal unit for their treatment.

Method: A retrospective review of retinal cases seen at the Eye Clinic of the University College Hospital, Ibadan, between 1998 and 2003, was carried out.

Results: 395 retinal cases were reviewed. Male to female ratio was 1.3:1. The peak age of presentation was 60 years and above. The common diseases noted were macular diseases (35.6%), comprising age-related macular degeneration (AMD), macular scar and holes. Retinochoroiditis (14.4%), retinitis pigmentosa (11.1%), retinal detachment (7.8%) and diabetic retinopathy (7.6%) were significant presentations. About 35.9% needed laser treatment, 20.8% needed vitreoretinal surgery, and 40% needed other vitreo-retinal investigations such as fundus fluorescein angiography.

Conclusion: The setting up of a vitreo-retinal unit is desirable at the University College Hospital, Ibadan.

2.   **Nazimul H, Rohit K, Taraprasad D, Raja N , Oluleye T, Azad G, Rajeev R, Two years follow-up outcome of verteporfin therapy for subfoveal choroidal neovascularization in pathologic myopia in Indian eyes.** *Ind. J. Ophth* **2008; 56: 465-8.**
Context: In India, refractive errors are a major cause of treatable blindness. Population surveys in southern India have shown the prevalence of high myopia to be 4.32-4.54%. Photodynamic therapy (PDT) for choroidal neovascularization (CNV) caused by pathologic myopia is beneficial.

Aim: To report the 24 months outcome of PDT with verteporfin for subfoveal CNV caused by pathologic myopia in Indian eyes.

Methodology: Review of prospectively collected data of Indian patients with pathologic myopia and subfoveal CNV treated with verteporfin therapy between 2001 and 2005, using a standard regimen for PDT.

Results: Fifteen patients (15 eyes) treated with standard fluence PDT and who had completed 24 months follow-up were analyzed. The mean spherical equivalent was -13.36 ± 5.88 diopter. Five out of 15 eyes in 6 months, 3 out of 15 eyes at 12 months and 4 eyes out of 15 at 24 months had improved vision by > 10 letters. The mean number of treatment session was 2.2 in two years.

Conclusions: PDT with verteporfin for subfoveal CNV caused by pathologic myopia in Indian eyes is effective.

Keywords: Choroidal neovascularization, pathologic myopia, photodynamic therapy, subfoveal, verteporfin.

3.   **Oluleye, TS. Age-related macular degeneration: Current concepts in pathogenesis and management. 2008; 16(1): 5-11.**

Age-related macular degeneration, which was once thought to be a disease mainly found among the Caucasian population in Europe and America, is now also appearing more frequently among non-white populations in the developing world. This paper reviews current concepts in the pathogenesis and management of age-related macular degeneration as found in Pubmed journals over the past ten years with a view to recommend optimal treatment regimens for African populations.

Keywords: Age-related macular degeneration, pathogenesis, genetics, management, anti-VEGF.

4.   **Oluleye TS, Ajayi O. Intravitreal triamcinolone in posterior segment diseases – Method of administration.** *Nig.J Oph,* **2009; 17(2): 74-76**

Intravitreal triamcinolone is indicated in the treatment of selected posterior segment disease. Method of administration is discussed. Post injection complications are also stressed.

5.   **Oluleye TS, Taiwo A. Ruptured retina artery macroaneurysm presenting with recurrent vitreous haemorrhage: A case report.** *Nig.J.Oph,* **2010; 18(1): 26**

A 74-year old hypertensive presented with recurrent vitreous haemorrhage. Examination showed a ruptured retinal arterial macroaneurysm. Control of systemic hypertension was associated with resolution. Risk factors and management are discussed. Ruptured retinal arterial macroaneurysm should be considered in elderly hypertensive patients presenting with vitreous haemorrhage.

Keywords: Retinal arterial macroaneurysm, vitreous haemorrhage, systemic hypertension.

6.   **Oluleye TS. Diabetic retinopathy: Current developments in pathogenesis and management.** *Afr J Med Med Sci.* **2010; 39(3): 199-206**

Diabetic retinopathy is now an important cause of visual impairment in the developing countries due to changing lifestyles. This review includes recent developments in the pathogenesis of diabetic retinopathy, emphasizing the role of protein kinase C and vascular endothelial growth factor. It also brings to the fore the atypical presentations, recent use of pharmacological agents and the importance of screening in the management of diabetic retinopathy. These developments are relevant in Nigeria, and ophthalmic and medical practitioners need to be aware.

7.   **Oluleye TS. Current management of diabetic maculopathy.** *J. Diabetes and Metabolism* **2011**

Diabetic maculopathy is a cause of significant visual loss in diabetic patients. Management of the condition focus on the presence of oedema or ischaemia. The role of laser and anti-VEGF is discussed.

8.   Oluleye TS. Best macular dystrophy in a Nigerian, a case report. *Case Rep Ophthalmol* **2012; 3: 205–208**

Best macular dystrophy is reported to be rare in Africans. It is a hereditary disease that starts in childhood and progresses through some stages before visual symptoms occur. This case report presents a 43-year old Nigerian with the disease and stresses the importance of regular eye exams of patients and relatives to detect changes such as choroidal neovascular membrane amenable to treatment.

Keywords: Best macular dystrophy, choroidal neovascular membrane, retina, Nigerian, tunnel vision.

9.   Oluleye T.S. Is age-related macular degeneration a problem in Ibadan, sub-Saharan Africa? *Clinical Ophthalmology* **2012; 6: 561–564**

Background: Age-related macular degeneration (AMD) is considered uncommon in black populations, including those of sub-Saharan Africa. The aim of this review was to determine the pattern of presentation of AMD in our hospital located in Ibadan, the largest city in sub-Saharan Africa.

Methods: A retrospective review of all cases with AMD presenting at the Eye and Retina Clinic of the University College Hospital, Ibadan, West Africa, was undertaken between October 2007 and September 2010.

Results: Seven hundred and sixty-eight retinal cases were seen in the hospital, 101 (14%) of which were diagnosed with AMD. The peak age was 60–79 years. The male to female ratio was approximately 2:3. More males presented with the advanced form of dry AMD than females (odds ratio = 2.33). However, more females had advanced wet AMD than males (odds ratio = 1.85). Wet AMD was seen in 40 cases (40%).

Conclusion: The review determined that, as AMD is not uncommon and wet AMD is relatively more common in our hospital than has been reported previously, this is probably true of Ibadan in general.

Keywords: Age-related maculopathy, choroidal neovascular membrane, retinal, vitreoretinal, drusen.

10.   Oluleye TS. Pattern of presentation of sickle cell retinopathy in Ibadan. *J Clinic Experiment Ophthalmol* **2012, 3: 257**

Background: Sickle cell retinopathy is not uncommon in Nigeria. Most cases of retinopathy occur in patients with the haemoglobin SC genotype. A significant proportion present late.

Methods: A review of 33 cases of sickle cell retinopathy seen over 3years (2008 - 2010) that presented at the Retina Unit of the Department of Ophthalmology, University College Hospital, Ibadan, were reviewed. Demographics and pattern of presentation were recorded in the proforma prepared for the study.

Results: Hb SC produces most of the presentations. The male: female ratio was 3:1. About two-thirds of the patients were below 40 years of age. Seventy percent of the patients presented with proliferative retinopathy. About half of them were blind at presentation. Pan retinal laser photocoagulation is the most common mode of treatment. The role of anti-VEGF intravitreal injection in the management of sickle cell retinopathy was discussed.

Conclusion: General/family physicians are to refer patients with sickle cell retinopathy for regular ophthalmic examinations to identify treatable lesions amenable to intervention.

Keywords: Sickle cell retinopathy, blindness, laser photocoagulation, anti-VEGF, screening

11.   **Oluleye TS. Should posterior vitrectomy be made a priority in ophthalmic facilities of sub-Saharan Africa?** *Open Ophthalmol J.* **2013; 7: 1-3**

Background: Posterior vitrectomy facilities are lacking in sub-Saharan Africa due to the paucity of trained personnel in the vitreretinal subspecialty. More cases are seen that require vitrectomy, especially cases with vitreous opacities and complications of cataract surgery, as more residents are being trained. The review will determine whether vitrectomy facility should be a priority as part of ophthalmic facilities in the region.

Method: A 3-year review was carried out. All cases of posterior vitrectomy performed at the Retina Unit of the University College Hospital, Ibadan, between 2008 and 2011, were retrieved. Indications and visual outcome were documented. Proportions and percentages were used to analyze the data.

Results: Sixty-six posterior vitrectomies were performed during the period. The most common indication for vitrectomy was vitreous haemorrhage (45.5%). Complications of cataract surgery such as dropped intraocular lens (10.7%), sclera fixated intra ocular lens (9.2%) and dropped nucleus (7.5%) were emerging indications. Other indications noted include complicated retinal detachments (6.1%), membranectomy for posterior capsule opacity from paediatric cataract surgery (4.5%) and congenital lens subluxation 2 (3.0%). Improved visual outcome was noted after surgery. Forty-nine (75%) eyes were blind (visual acuity of < 3/60) before vitrectomy. This proportion dropped to 24 (37%) after vitrectomy, with an additional 24% regaining navigational vision (visual acuity of 3/60 to counting fingers at 1m) .

Conclusion: Vitrectomy should be an integral part of eye care and its availability should be made a priority in ophthalmic facilities of sub-Saharan Africa, especially those involved in ophthalmology training.

Keywords: Cataract surgery complications, posterior vitrectomy, retinal, sub-Saharan Africa, vitreous opacities.

12.   **Oluleye TS. Tuberculous uveitis.** *Journal of Multidisciplinary Healthcare* **2013; 6: 41-3**.

Tuberculous uveitis is an under-diagnosed form of uveitis. Absence of pulmonary signs and symptoms does not rule out the disease. In an era of reduced immunity from human immunodeficiency virus and acquired immunodeficiency syndrome, the disease is becoming more prevalent. This review discusses the common manifestations of tuberculous uveitis, pointing out helpful diagnostic criteria in suspicious cases of uveitis. Physicians need to be aware that ocular manifestations of tuberculosis may be independent of systemic disease.

Keywords: tuberculous uveitis, ocular manifestations, tuberculosis.

13.   **Oluleye TS, Aina AS, Sarimiye TF, Olaniyan SI. Stagardt's disease in 2 Nigerian siblings.** *International Medical Case Report Journal* **2013. 6: 13-15**

Stargardt's disease is an inherited macular dystrophy that is transmitted in an autosomal recessive or dominant pattern. The disorder is typically characterized by impairment of central vision, with onset around the first 10–20 years of life. Stargardt's disease is rare in sub-Saharan Africa. This is probably the first reported case in the subregion. We present two siblings with the disease. Presentation, pathophysiology and management modalities are discussed.

Keywords: Stargardt's disease, macular dystrophy, retinal, Nigerians

14.   **Oluleye TS, Babalola Y. Pattern of presentation of idiopathic polypoidal choroidal vasculopathy in Ibadan, sub-Saharan Africa.** *Clinical Ophthalmology* **2013; 7: 1373-6**

Background: Idiopathic polypoidal choroidal vasculopathy is an abnormal choroidal vascular pathology similar to age-related macular degeneration. It may present with sudden visual loss from haemorrhagic retinal pigment epithelial detachment and breakthrough vitreous haemorrhage or with chronic recurrent episodes. The condition is not uncommon in the retina clinic at the University College Hospital, Ibadan, sub-Saharan Africa. This study presents the pattern of presentation in Ibadan.

Methods: We review all cases of idiopathic polypoidal choroidal vasculopathy seen from 2007 to 2012 at the Retina Clinic of the University College Hospital, Ibadan, to determine the major pattern of presentations, available treatment modalities and visual outcomes.

Results: Ten cases were seen during the study period. Their mean age was 58 years, with a male to female ratio of 1:4. The most common presenting complaint was sudden visual loss. Major examination findings were retinal pigment epithelial detachment, orange subretinal lesions and breakthrough vitreous haemorrhage. The modalities of treatment available include vitrectomy to clear vitreous haemorrhage. Intravitreal bevacizumab reduced the height of the pigment epithelial detachment and cleared vitreous haemorrhage. Thermal laser was applied for extrafoveal lesions. Two patients with subfoveal lesions were referred abroad for photodynamic therapy. Visual outcome showed significant improvement in vitrectomized patients who presented with vitreous haemorrhage. Presenting vision of hand motion and light perception improved vision ranging from counting fingers to 6/12 after vitrectomy.

Conclusion: Idiopathic polypoidal choroidal vasculopathy may not be uncommon in sub-Saharan Africa. A high index of suspicion is warranted in the diagnosis so as to provide timely intervention.

Keywords: Idiopathic polypoidal choroidal vasculopathy, retinal pigment epithelial detachment, presentations, sub-Saharan Africa.

15.   Oluleye TS, Ibrahim O, Olusanya B. Scleral buckling for retinal detachment in Ibadan, sub-Saharan Africa: Anatomical and visual outcome. *Clinical Ophthalmol.* **2013; 7: 1049-52**

Background: Scleral buckle surgery is not a commonly performed surgical procedure in sub-Saharan Africa due to a paucity of trained vitreoretinal surgeons. The aim of the study was to review sclera buckle procedures with a view to evaluating the anatomical and visual outcomes.

Methods: Case records of patients that had scleral buckle surgery at the Retina Unit of the University College Hospital, Ibadan, Nigeria, between 2007 and 2010, were reviewed. The information retrieved include patients' demographics, duration of symptoms, presenting vision, site of retinal break, extent of retinal detachment, involvement of the fellow eye and macular involvement. Postoperative retina reattachment and postoperative visual acuity were also recorded. Proportions and percentages were used to analyze the data.

Results: Forty-five eyes of 42 patients were studied, with a male to female ratio of 1.6:1. The mean age was 47.7 years (±17.6 years). The median duration before presentation was 3 months (range: 5 days – 156 months). Subtotal retinal detachment was found in 35 eyes (77.8%), while total retinal detachment occurred in 10 eyes (22.2%). Thirty-four eyes (75.6%) had 'macular off' detachments. At 6 weeks, there was an improvement in visual acuity in 23 eyes (51.1%), while visual acuity remained the same in 9 eyes (20%) and was worse in 13 eyes (28.9%). Anatomical attachment was seen in 43 eyes (95.6%) on the operation table, in 40 eyes (90.9%) at first day postoperatively and in 32 eyes (86.5%) at 6 weeks after surgery.

Conclusion: Outcome of sclera buckle surgery for rhegmatogenous retinal detachment may be improved in developing countries of sub-Saharan Africa if adequate awareness is created to educate the populace on early presentation.

Keywords: Retinal detachment, scleral buckle surgery, anatomical and visual outcomes, Ibadan.

16.   Oluleye TS, Babalola Y. Indications for intravitreal bevacizumab in Ibadan, sub-Saharan Africa. *Open Ophthalmology Journal* **2014; 8: 87-90**

Background: Angiogenesis is a contributing factor in some retinal diseases, hence the role of vascular endothelial growth factor (VEGF) as a common pathway in proliferative retinopathies. Bevacizumab has been found to be effective in the treatment of these diseases. The aim of this study was to review all cases of intravitreal bevacizumab given at the Retina Unit of the University College Hospital, Ibadan, from July 2010 to June 2012, pointing out the common indications.

Methods: After obtaining ethical approval from the University College Hospital/University of Ibadan Review Board for the study, all cases of intravitreal injections of bevacizumab recorded in the retinal register during the study period (July 2010 to June 2012) were retrieved. Age, sex, diagnoses and indication for injection were recorded in the data sheet prepared for the study. Results were analyzed using proportions and percentages.

Results: A total of 134 injections of bevacizumab were given during the study period. The most common indication was cystoid macular oedema from retinal vein occlusion (19.4%), followed by wet age-related maculopathy (17.1%) and sickle cell retinopathy (16.4). Emerging indications include idiopathic polypoidal choroidal vasculopathy (6%) and retinal macroaneurism with macular oedema (4.5%).

Conclusion: Cystoid macular oedema from vascular occlusion and wet age-related macular degeneration are the major indications for intravitreal bevacizumab injection in Ibadan.

Keywords: Cystoid macular oedema, intravitreal bevacizumab, retinal vein occlusion, sickle cell retinopathy.

17.   **Oluleye TS. Mobile phones for fundus photography in Ibadan, sub-Saharan Africa.** *Advances in Ophthalmology and Visual Sciences* **2014; 1(4): 00020(1-3)**

Background: Fundus photography is essential for documentation, patient education and monitoring follow-up treatments in patients with retinal diseases. The equipment for fundus photography is expensive for most ophthalmic facilities in sub-Saharan Africa. Mobile technology is a cheaper alternative, as this will enhance telemedical services in the region.

Aim: The aim of this study was to investigate the use of Iphone 5 in combination with a 20D lens to capture retinal images. The Iphone 5 was also compared with the cheaper android phone, Techno phantom A+.

Methods: We selected consecutive patients attending the Retina Clinic of the University College Hospital, Ibadan, for the study. Informed consent was obtained before the study. Five patients each with retinal diseases affecting the posterior pole within the field of view of the 20D lens were enrolled to either Iphone 5 plus 20D lens or Techno A+ plus 20D lens after full pupillary dilatation. The setup is used as a binocular indirect ophthalmoscope. The eye of the patient, the 20D lens and the flash/camera of the mobile phone must be on the same axis. The 20D lens captures the image of the retina, which is viewed by the examiner on the screen of the mobile phone. The application, Filmic Pro, improves the stability of image capturing of the Iphone system. The two systems were compared for ease of use, resolution and clarity of pictures.

Results: The Iphone 5 system and the Techno system showed comparable results. The Iphone 5 produced fewer glare with clearer pictures.

Conclusion: The mobile technology described is a cheaper alternative to standard fundus photography in sub-Saharan Africa.

Keywords: Mobile phones, fundus photography, retinal disease, patient education, telemedicine, sub-Saharan Africa.

18.   **Oluleye TS, Olusanya B. Barriers to setting up a vitreoretinal unit of ophthalmology in Ibadan, sub-Saharan Africa.** *Nigerian Journal of Ophthalmology* **2014; 22(2): 95-96**

The challenges of setting up of a vitreoretinal centre in Ibadan is discussed. The possibility of overcoming the challenges was highlighted.

19.   **Adeoye AM, Oluleye TS, Olusanya BA. PM248 association of left ventricular wall thickness and retinopathy among patients with essential hypertension.** *Global Heart* 2014; 9(Supplement 1): e111-e11

Introduction: In a nested case–control analysis of the Beaver Dam Eye Study, individuals with hypertensive retinopathy were twice as likely to die from cardiovascular events as those without these signs. An earlier study from Asia showed no significant relationship between LVH severity and retinopathy. There is a dearth of data among subjects of African descent. We report the association between left ventricular relative wall thickness and hypertensive retinopathy.

Objectives: To assess the association between left ventricular relative wall thickness and hypertensive retinopathy.

Methods: One hundred and fifty-six consecutive newly-presenting hypertensives (73 males and 83 females) with informed consent were recruited for the study. All participants underwent full clinical evaluation and echocardiographic examination was performed according to the ASE recommendation. The degree of retinopathy on ophthalmological examination was defined according to the Keith-Wagener classification. Left ventricular hypertrophy was considered present if the left ventricular mass index is greater than or equal to $51g/m^2$. Relative wall thickness (RWT) was calculated as 2PWTd/LVIDd. Increased wall thickness was present when RWT >0.45. Left ventricular geometry was stratified using left ventricular mass index and relative wall thickness.

Results: The mean age of the hypertensive subjects was 59.5 (12.3) years. Ocular examination revealed normal (20.9%), grade I retinopathy 45.1%), grade II retinopathy (32.0%) and grade III retinopathy (1.3%). There is a positive correlation between LV relative wall thickness and severity of retinopathy in both eyes. There was no correlation between LV geometric pattern and retinopathy.

Conclusion: The study showed a strong positive relation between LV relative wall thickness and grades of retinopathy. This study suggests a simultaneous target organ damage associated with hypertension. Prompt management of hypertension in the study population may prevent untoward cardiovascular events.

20.   **Oluleye TS, Rotimi-Samuel A, Adenekan A. Mobile phones for retinopathy of prematurity screening in Lagos, Nigeria, sub-Saharan Africa.** *Eur J Ophthalmol.* 2016; 26(1): 92-4

Aim: Retinopathy of prematurity (ROP), thought to be rare in Nigeria, sub-Saharan Africa, has been reported in recent studies. Developing cost-effective screening is crucial for detecting retinal changes amenable to treatment. This study describes the use of an Iphone combined with a 20-D lens in screening for ROP in Lagos, Nigeria.

Methods: The ROP screening programme was approved by the Lagos University Teaching Hospital Ethical Committee. Preterm infants with birth weight of less than 1.5 kg or gestational age of less than 32 weeks were screened. In conjunction with the neonatologist, topical tropicamide (0.5%) and phenylephrine (2.5%) were used to dilate the pupils. A paediatric lid speculum was used. Indirect ophthalmoscopy was used to examine the fundus to ensure there were no missed diagnoses. An Iphone 5 with 20-D lens was used to examine the fundus. The app, Filmic Pro, was launched in the video mode. The camera flash served as the source of illumination. Its intensity was controlled by the app. The 20-D lens was used to capture the image of the retina, which was picked up by the camera system of the mobile phone. Another app, Aviary, was used to edit the picture.

Results: The images captured by the system were satisfactory for staging and determining the need for treatment.

Conclusion: An Iphone combined with a 20-D lens appear to be useful in screening for ROP in resource-poor settings. More studies are needed in this area.

21.   **Oluleye TS, Babalola Y, Ijaduola M. Chloroquine retinopathy: Pattern of presentation in Ibadan.** *Eye (Lond)* **2016; 30(1): 64-7**

Background: Self-medication with chloroquine is common in Ibadan, sub-Saharan Africa. Retinopathy from chloroquine is not uncommon. The aim was to determine the pattern of presentation.

Methodology: Cases of chloroquine retinopathy seen at the Retina and Vitreous Unit of the University College Hospital, Ibadan, between 2008 and 2014, were reviewed. Information on age, sex, duration of chloroquine use and visual loss were retrieved. Visual acuity at presentation, anterior and posterior segment findings were documented. The results were analyzed using proportions and percentages.

Results: Fourteen cases were seen during the study period. Mean age was 50.7 years. The male to female ratio was 3.5:1. The average duration of visual loss before presentation was 2.7 years. The average duration of self-medication with chloroquine was 5.3 years. Presenting visual acuity showed 2 cases of bilateral blindness (VA<3/60 in both eyes), 5 cases of uniocular blindness and 3 cases of bilateral low vision (VA worse than 6/18 but better than 3/60). Anterior segment examination showed abnormal sluggish pupillary reaction in those with severe affectation. Dilated fundoscopy showed features ranging from mild macular pigmentary changes and bulls eye maculopathy to overt extensive retinal degeneration involving the posterior pole, attenuation of retinal vessels, optic atrophy and beaten bronze appearance of atrophic maculopathy.

Conclusion: Chloroquine retinopathy is not uncommon in Ibadan, sub-Saharan Africa. Bulls eye maculopathy, extensive retinal and macular degeneration with optic atrophy are the main presentations. Public health education is imperative.

22.   **Olusanya BA, Oluleye TS. Unilateral central serous chorioretinopathy in a pregnant Nigerian woman.** *Nig. Med. Journal* **2015; 56(5): 372-374**

Central serous chorioretinopathy (CSCR) is an idiopathic condition characterized by serous detachment of the neurosensory retina in the macular region. It is relatively uncommon in Africans and though pregnancy is a known risk factor, there are no previous reports of CSCR in pregnant African women. We reported the case of a 35-year old pregnant woman who presented to our clinic at gestational age of 29 weeks, with a 4 months history of blurring of vision in her left eye. Examination revealed visual acuity of 6/4 on the right eye and 6/9 on the left eye. She had normal anterior segments bilaterally and a normal posterior segment on the right. However, she had left macular oedema with exudates. There was no significant refractive error. Her blood pressure was normal. Investigations including electrolytes and urea, urinalysis and blood sugar profile were all normal. She was managed conservatively and symptoms resolved 2 weeks prior to delivery. Pregnant women should be educated about the possibility of visual problems accompanying pregnancy.

Keywords: Nigeria, ocular manifestations, pregnancy.

23.   **Ibrahim OA, Foster A, Oluleye TS. Barriers to an effective diabetic retinopathy service in Ibadan, Nigeria (sub –Saharan Africa).** *Ann Ibd. Pg. Med* **2015; 13(1): 36-43**

Background: Diabetic retinopathy is an increasing cause of blindness. The prevalence of retinopathy in hospital-attending diabetics in Ibadan is reported to be 42 %. This study assessed the barriers identified by patients and service providers to delivering good services for diabetic retinopathy in Ibadan, Nigeria, sub-Saharan Africa.

Methods: A qualitative survey using non-participatory observation, in-depth interviews (patients and healthcare providers) and focus group discussion for diabetic patients in the eye clinic in the University College Hospital, Ibadan, was done. A semi-structured interview and topic guides were used to evaluate the barriers to effective service. The participants were selected using a non-probability, purposive sampling strategy. Twenty participants were involved in the pilot study. There were ten in-depth interviews of patients and two focus group discussions of patients (3 in each group). Four healthcare providers were interviewed (a retinal surgeon, a senior registrar, an endocrinologist and a public health nurse).

Results: Lack of awareness that diabetes causes irreversible blindness was identified as a major barrier by both patients and providers. Cost of treatment of diabetes and treatment of retinopathy was also an important barrier. The long waiting time before consultation, staff attitudes to patients and appointment scheduling problems deterred patients from using the service.

Conclusion: More diabetic patients can be encouraged by providing more detailed information/counselling and making clinic attendance less costly and more convenient.

Keywords: Barriers, diabetic retinopathy, service, Ibadan.

24.   **Oluleye ST, Olusanya BA, Adeoye AM. Retinal vascular changes in hypertensive patients in Ibadan, sub-Saharan Africa.** *Int J Gen Med.* **2016; 9: 285-90**

Background: Earlier studies in Nigeria reported the rarity of retinal vascular changes in hypertensives. The aim of this study was to describe the various retinal vascular changes in the hypertensive patients of Nigeria.

Methods: Nine hundred and three hypertensive patients were studied. This study was approved by the ethical and research committee of the University of Ibadan and University College Hospital, Ibadan, Nigeria. Blood pressure and anthropometric measurements were measured. Cardiac echocardiography was performed on 156 patients. All patients had dilated fundoscopy and fundus photography using the Kowa portable fundus camera and an Apple Iphone with 20 D lens. Statistical analysis was carried by the Statistical Packages for the Social Sciences (Version 21).

Results: The mean age of patients was 57 years, with a male: female ratio of 1. No retinopathy was found in 556 (61.5%) patients. In all, 175 (19.4%) patients had features of hypertensive retinopathy. Retinal vascular occlusion was a significant finding in 121 patients (13.4%), of which branch retinal vein occlusion (4.7%) and central retinal vein occlusion (3.3%) were the most prominent ones in cases. Hemicentral retinal vein occlusion (2.9%) and central retinal artery occlusion (1.9%) were significant presentations. Other findings include nonarteritic anterior ischaemic optic neuropathy (0.6%), hypertensive choroidopathy (0.8%) and haemorrhagic choroidal detachment (0.6%). Left ventricular (LV) geometry was abnormal in 85 (55.5%) patients. Concentric remodeling, eccentric hypertrophy and concentric hypertrophy were observed in 43 (27.6%), 26 (17.2%) and 15 (9.7%) patients, respectively. LV hypertrophy was found in 42 (27%) patients, while 60 (39%) patients had increased relative wall thickness. In this study, bivariate analysis showed a correlation between LV relative wall thickness and severity of retinopathy in both eyes (Spearman's coefficient 0.6; P=0.0004).

Conclusion: Hypertensive retinal vascular changes are not rare in Ibadan.

Keywords: Hypertensive retinopathy, retinal vascular occlusion, retinal vascular changes, left ventricular wall thickness, Ibadan.

25. **Onakpoya OH, Adeoti CO, Oluleye TS, Ajayi IA, Majengbasan T, Olorundare OK. Clinical presentation and visual status of retinitis pigmentosa patients: A multicenter study in southwestern Nigeria.** *Clinical Ophthalmology* **2016: 10: 1579-1583**

Background: To review the visual status and clinical presentation of patients with retinitis pigmentosa (RP).

Methodology: A multicentre, retrospective and analytical review of the visual status and clinical characteristics of patients with RP at first presentation from January 2007 to December 2011, was conducted. Main outcome measure was the World Health Organization's visual status classification in relation to sex and age at presentation. Data analysis carried out by SPSS (version 15) and statistical significance was assumed at P<0.05.

Results: One hundred and ninety-two eyes of 96 patients, with a mean age of 39.08±18.5 years and mode of 25 years constituted the study population. Fifty-five (57.3%) of the patients were male and 41 (42.7%) were female. Loss of vision (69.8%) and night blindness (58.3%) were the leading symptoms. Twenty-one (21.9%) patients had a positive family history, with RP present in their siblings (71.4%), grandparents (52.3%) and parents (19.4%). Forty (41.7%) were blind at presentation and 23 (24%) were visually impaired. Blindness in 6(15%) patients was secondary to glaucoma. Retinal vascular narrowing and retinal pigmentary changes of varying severity were present in all patients. Thirty-five (36.5%) had maculopathy, 36 (37.5%) had refractive error, 19(20%) had lenticular opacities and 11(11.5%) had glaucoma. Retinitis pigmentosa was typical in 85 (88.5%) patients. Older patients had higher rates of blindness at presentation (P=0.005). Blindness and visual impairment rate at presentation were higher in the males patients than in the female patients (P=0.029).

Conclusion: Clinical presentation with advanced diseases, higher blindness rate in older patients, sex-related difference in blindness/visual impairment rates, as well as high glaucoma blindness in RP patients requires urgent attention in southwestern Nigeria.

Keywords: Retinitis pigmentosa, blindness, glaucoma, visual impairment, Nigeria.

26.   Oluleye TS, Brown BJ, Olawoye O. Ocular manifestations of children with sickle cell disease in Ibadan, Nigeria. *East African Medical Journal* **2017; 94(10): 812-819**

Background: Children with sickle cell disease can present with ocular complaints. Regular eye examination can detect sight threatening conditions amenable to treatment. The aim of the study was to describe ocular manifestations of children with sickle cell disease attending the Paediatric Outpatient Department of the University College Hospital, Ibadan.

Methodology: Children 15 years and below diagnosed with the sickle cell disease at the Paediatric Outpatient of the University College Hospital were examined in detail by the ophthalmologist to document ocular findings.

Results: One hundred and five patients were examined. The mean age was 3.22 ± 2.49 years, with a male to female ratio of 1.2: 1. Ninety (85.7%) children had haemoglobin SS, while 15(14.3%) had HB SC. The important ocular findings were retinal vascular tortuosity in 15(14.3%) patients, central retinal artery occlusion in 2(1.9%) patients, black sunbursts pigmentation in 2(1.9%) patients, chorioretinal atrophy in 3(2.8%) patients, salmon patch retina haemorrhage in 1(0.95%) patient, retina holes in 1(0.95%) patient and retina coloboma in 1(0.95%) patient. The only anterior segment finding was jaundice in all the patients. No conjunctiva vascular abnormalities were found.

Conclusion: Retinal vascular tortuosity is the most common ocular manifestation of children with sickle cell disease in Ibadan. Central retinal artery occlusion, a devastating condition, is an emerging manifestation. Regular eye examination for sickle cell retinopathy in children less than 15 years of age is not recommended.

27.   Fiebai B, Oluleye TS, Omaka IO. Coats disease in Nigeria: A case series. *Asian Journal of Medicine and Health* **2018; 13(3): 1-6**

Aim: To report a series of four cases of Coats disease in black Nigerians.

Study design: A case series.

Place and duration of study: The Retina Unit of the Departments of ophthalmology of the University College Hospital, Ibadan, Oyo State and the University of Port Harcourt Teaching Hospital, Rivers State, Nigeria. The duration of study was 2014-2018.

Methodology: Case folders of patients who presented at the Retina Units of the University College Hospital, Ibadan, University of Port Harcourt Teaching Hospital and a peripheral eye hospital, between 2014 and 2018, were reviewed. Data collected include age, sex, presenting visual acuity, findings on fundus examination and reports of ancillary tests.

Results: Four eyes of 4 patients were reviewed. There were 2 males and 2 females. Three of the 4 cases were found in children, while one case presented in adulthood. All eyes presented with profound visual loss, with uniocular presentation, exudative retinal detachments at the late stages and poor visual prognosis.

Conclusion: Coat's disease, though an uncommon ocular disorder in Nigeria, does exist and may have been underdiagnosed or misdiagnosed. Routine examination of children is pertinent in early diagnosis and prompt treatment to save vision. A good knowledge of its clinical presentation may lead to more case findings.

28.   **Ademola-Popoola DS, Oluleye TS. Retinopathy of prematurity (ROP) in a developing economy with improving health care.** *Current Ophthalmology Reports* **2017; 5(2): 114–118**

The aim of this study was to highlight the changing pattern of retinopathy of prematurity (ROP) incidence, with improvement in economy and health care in Africa, pointing out the challenges and recommendations for sustainable, cost-effective screening and management. Retinopathy of prematurity was initially thought to be rare in some parts of Africa. Recent findings have shown this not to be true.

Studies done in 2011–2016 reported the presence of any ROP stage in 12–52% of screened babies, with the prevalence of treatable ROP at 2.9–9.8%. ROP-trained ophthalmologists available to screen with binocular indirect ophthalmoscope and manage babies are few. Awareness of this blinding disease, disease screening, adequate follow-up, treatment issues, and physician competing duties are the major factors militating against effective ROP programmes.

Creating awareness and collaboration among stakeholders is urgently needed in most parts of Africa. Cost-effective, regional ROP screening programmes across several contiguous states using a telemedicine approach with widefield retinal imaging by middle level personnel is strongly advocated to best address the growing problem of ROP in many parts of Africa.

29.   **Olusanya BA, Oluleye TS, Tongo OO, Ugalahi MO,Babalola YO, Ayede AI, Baiyeroju AM. Retinopathy of prematurity in a tertiary facility: An initial report of a screening programme.** *Niger J Paediatr* **2020; 47(2): 55–60**

Aim: Retinopathy of prematurity (ROP) screening in Nigeria is at a nascent stage and, at the moment, there are no national guidelines for ROP screening in Nigeria. Thus, it is desirable for screening programmes to report findings amongst screened preterm infants in order to facilitate the development of a national ROP screening criteria and guidelines. The aim of this report was to describe the frequency, severity and risk factors for retinopathy of prematurity (ROP) among preterm and very low-birth-weight babies screened within the first year of initiating an ROP screening programme at a Nigerian tertiary facility.

Methods: A cross-sectional study of infants born at less than 34 weeks gestational age, or with birth weight less than 1500g, between May 2016 and May 2017, was conducted. ROP screening examinations were performed by ophthalmologists with the use of an indirect ophthalmoscope, after pupillary dilation, in collaboration with the neonatology team. Information on gestational age at birth, birth weight, oxygen therapy and presence of other risk factors were recorded and analyzed.

Results: A total of 74 infants were screened during the period. There were 36(48.6%) males. The mean gestational age at birth was 29.6 (±2.35) weeks. The mean birth weight was 1.26 (±0.27)kg, with a range of 800 to 1950g. ROP was detected in 9(12.2%) infants. Two (22.2%) of these had threshold ROP. There was no significant difference between the mean birth weight and mean gestational age of the infants who had ROP compared to those without ROP. The two infants with threshold ROP were treated with intravitreal bevazicumab and had regression of ROP.

Conclusion: Retinopathy of prematurity was diagnosed in at risk infants in this facility. There is, therefore, a need to establish ROP screening programmes in all neonatal units across the country. In addition, established programmes need to evaluate their screening criteria with a
view towards developing country-specific screening guidelines.

Index

Printed in the United States
By Bookmasters